Praise fo.
Bumpin'

A National Parenting Product Award Winner

"*Bumpin'* is like having your pregnancy best friend on call. It's not a quick-fix book that makes you feel stupid—Leslie Schrock has written the guide for the modern parent who is sick of being scared by the internet and wants a trusted resource."

—Lora Shahine, MD, FACOG, reproductive endocrinologist
at Pacific NW Fertility, and host of *Baby or Bust* podcast

"Leslie Schrock covers it all! As mothers of singletons followed by twins, we found *Bumpin'* to be full of important information that will help so many women who are already or hoping to become pregnant. The data is provided in a complete but compassionate and readable way, and the personal stories provide powerful firsthand advice. This book supports women through every stage of the family-planning process: from trying to become pregnant (including those with fertility issues), through pregnancy, and the postpartum phase."

—Rachel Brem, MD, and Christy Teal, MD, coauthors of
*No Longer Radical: Understanding Mastectomies
and Choosing the Breast Cancer Care That's Right for You*

"Every parent-to-be should own this book. As a mom of two, registered dietitian, and author, I can tell you that Leslie Schrock covers every question I had and those I wish I knew to ask. *Bumpin'* is an incredibly thorough, trustworthy, and easily digestible guide."

—Stephanie Middleberg, MS, RD, CDN, bestselling author of *The Big Book of Pregnancy Nutrition, The Big Book of Organic Baby Food*, and *The Big Book of Organic Toddler Food*, and founder of Middleberg Nutrition

"Leslie Schrock has done pregnant people and their partners a tremendous service with this book. Written with warmth, candor, and scientific rigor, *Bumpin'* is an essential guide to navigating the time before, during, and after pregnancy. I especially appreciated the new chapter on exercise, which promises to help readers move through pregnancy and beyond feeling as strong, steady, and pain-free as possible."

—Danielle Friedman, author of *Let's Get Physical:
How Women Discovered Exercise and Reshaped the World*

"*Bumpin'* belongs on every parent's nightstand; the best friend every new mother (and father) needs. As a mother of three and investor in women's and family health, I turn to Leslie and *Bumpin'* for clear, evidence-based, no-nonsense, and up-to-date answers to pressing questions. The latest edition makes this classic even more timely."

—Deena Shakir, investor and author of *Leena Mo, CEO*

"Behold a pregnancy and early-motherhood book that doesn't feel like a long and winding lecture. . . . So many moms and influencers . . . recommend this guide for expecting parents since it takes an unstuffy science-backed approach to insights."

—*Glamour* magazine

"A smart, approachable guide packed with practical advice for parents who want a science-backed, individualized approach to pregnancy."

—Linda Avey, cofounder of 23andMe

"Tech investor and new mom Leslie Schrock offers a thoroughly modern guide to pregnancy—from the preparations of 'trimester zero' to the challenges of the newborn months. With the frank, funny warmth of a trusted friend, she delves into everything from in vitro fertilization and prenatal testing to lactation consultants, debunking pregnancy myths and citing the latest science to help you make the best decisions every step of the way—for both you and your baby."

—National Parenting Product Awards

"Expectant millennial moms are hailing this book as the 'new pregnancy bible' and 'the only pregnancy book you need.' Leslie Schrock walks readers through what she's identified as the five trimesters of pregnancy, from pre-conception through the first few months with [your] baby, debunking myths with the latest scientific data and offering empathetic guidance with a healthy dose of real talk."

—The Bump

Praise for
Fertility Rules

"Leslie Schrock has created a practical, deeply researched guide that combines published clinical data with practical advice, using food as the framework to help everyone prepare for conception and pregnancy. *Fertility Rules* proves once again that food truly is medicine, especially when it comes to maximizing fertility."

—Mark Hyman, MD, *New York Times* bestselling
author of *The Pegan Diet*

"This is a much-needed book. . . . Schrock's coverage lives up to the promise of the subtitle. This is a definitive and highly useful guide to reproductive health."

—*Booklist* (starred review)

"From basics of the menstrual cycle to detailed guide on fertility optimization—this book has it all. Whether you just want to learn more about reproductive health or you're looking for ways to advocate for your fertility care—you've got it in *Fertility Rules*."

—Lora Shahine, MD, FACOG, reproductive endocrinologist
at Pacific NW Fertility, and host of *Baby or Bust* podcast

Revised & Expanded Second Edition

bumpin'

Navigating the Wild, Weird, and Wonderful Journey Through Pregnancy from Conception to Birth and Beyond

leslie schrock

Medical editor: Jane van Dis, MD: Obstetrics/Gynecology

Simon Element

New York   Amsterdam/Antwerp   London
Toronto   Sydney   New Delhi

SIMON ELEMENT

An Imprint of Simon & Schuster, LLC
1230 Avenue of the Americas
New York, NY 10020

This Simon Element trade paperback edition March 2025

SIMON ELEMENT is a trademark of Simon & Schuster, LLC

This publication contains the opinions and ideas of its author. It is intended to provide helpful and informative material on the subjects addressed in the publication. It is sold with the understanding that the author and publisher are not engaged in rendering medical, health, or any other kind of personal professional services in the book. The reader should consult his or her medical, health, or other competent professional before adopting any of the suggestions in this book or drawing inferences from it. The author and publisher specifically disclaim all responsibility for any liability, loss, or risk, personal or otherwise, which is incurred as a consequence, directly or indirectly, of the use and application of any of the contents of this book.

For information about special discounts for bulk purchases, please contact Simon & Schuster Special Sales at 1-866-506-1949 or business@simonandschuster.com.

The Simon & Schuster Speakers Bureau can bring authors to your live event. For more information or to book an event, contact the Simon & Schuster Speakers Bureau at 1-866-248-3049 or visit our website at www.simonspeakers.com.

Manufactured in the United States of America

10 9 8 7 6 5 4 3 2 1

Library of Congress Cataloging-in-Publication Data
Names: Schrock, Leslie, author.
Title: Bumpin : navigating the wild, weird, and wonderful journey through pregnancy from conception to birth and beyond / Leslie Schrock ;
   Medical editor, Jane van Dis, MD: Obstetrics/Gynecology.
Description: Revised & expanded second edition. | New York : Simon Element,
   2025. | Includes bibliographical references and index.
Identifiers: LCCN 2024020199 | ISBN 9781668050118 | ISBN 9781982130459 (ebook)
Subjects: LCSH: Pregnancy—Popular works. | Motherhood—Popular works.
Classification: LCC RG525 .S375 2025 | DDC 618.2—dc23/eng/20240906
LC record available at https://lccn.loc.gov/2024020199

ISBN 978-1-6680-5011-8
ISBN 978-1-9821-3045-9 (ebook)

To Mr. Baby—you were worth the wait.
And to Nick, who was by my side through it all.

It's no use going back to yesterday,
because I was a different person then.

—Lewis Carroll, *Alice's Adventures in Wonderland*

Contents

Foreword to the Second Edition   **xiii**

Preface   **xvii**

Trimester Zero   **1**

Get Ready   3

Making a Baby   21

If Things Get Bumpy   33

The First Trimester   **49**

Pregnancy FAQ, Lightning Round   63

Your Care Team Fantasy Draft   77

Things to Avoid   95

Pregnant Bodies Are Strong Bodies   111

To Test or Not to Test?   133

The Second Trimester   **147**

What Do I Actually Need to Buy?   157

Meet Your Pelvic Floor   167

It's Not a Birth *Plan*—It's Preferences   175

The Third Trimester   **201**

    Life Right Before—and After—Birth   213

    The Big Event   235

The Fourth Trimester   **261**

    Recovery   281

    Feeding Time   297

    Your New Roommate   325

    Transitions   337

Acknowledgments   **347**

Bibliography   **349**

Index   **369**

FOREWORD TO THE SECOND EDITION

It's been five years since the publication of *Bumpin'*, and as a practicing ob-gyn and professor of obstetrics and gynecology, I can honestly say that nothing has brought me more joy than seeing expecting parents find answers to their questions. Many readers have even gone deeper into the primary sources I assisted Leslie Schrock in compiling as her medical editor. In revisiting this second edition, I was struck once more by Leslie's effervescent, uncensored warmth. I hope this reissue, updated with expanded information and sources, continues the legacy of the first edition, which made accessible the insider medical information and truths that should guide your decisions. Every pregnant woman deserves that.

From the patient's perspective, the practice of obstetrics may not feel as collaborative as we would like, partly because we don't always do the best job of talking across our respective aisles but also because there are thousands of information sources for women to turn to today. What I haven't seen is a book that combines the rigor and precision of the best medical literature with the wisdom of specialists from various disciplines, training, and backgrounds—and delivers it with the expert reassurance of personal experience. In this book, Leslie Schrock has done just that, not only for the process of pregnancy itself but also for fertility, conception, and all things postpartum.

The practice of obstetrics evolves more slowly than other fields for reasons ranging from the challenges of performing randomized controlled trials on a mother-fetal cohort, the dramatic physiological changes that happen during pregnancy, ethical considerations around safety, fear of the maternal body, and a light sprinkling of misogyny. Obstetrics is a daunting profession, too. Unlike in any other medical specialty, there are two patients—two hearts asynchronously beating and two sets of expectations, both fragile and intertwined. Not to mention familial and cultural inheritances that often go well beyond those two lives.

Obstetrics is so much more than facts in a medical school textbook. The wisdom that many doctors bring to obstetrics comes from a range of sources: midwives who have shared expertise on maternal positions in labor; maternal-fetal medicine specialists who contextualize complex genetic abnormalities or fetal malformations; doulas who demonstrate how to center the pregnant woman in her particular narrative; labor nurses whose wisdom, laughter, advocacy, and sheer tenacity keep us sane day after day. And let's be honest: carrying my twins and becoming a mother certainly taught me a thing or two. Obstetrics is a team sport.

In medicine, we contend with physiological limits: blood pressure and heart rates, hormones, and neurotransmitters. With the architecture of birth, the bones of the maternal pelvis can expand only so much. With physics, a uterus has only so much power to push the infant out against opposing forces. And with the senses, a maternal body can withstand only a finite amount of pain.

With all the technology available to us, it's easy to forget that the process of pregnancy and birth is a mixture of physiology, environment, mostly genetics, and a bit of the unexplained and random. We can treat things like preterm labor and preeclampsia when they occur, but we are less adept at predicting to whom those things will happen and instead rely on risk factors and demographics. I am consistently surprised that healthy women can sometimes have the most complicated pregnancies, and women with serious risk factors can avoid any complications at all. *Bumpin'* has been updated to help women understand when to seek help. And of course, I understand that for women, the process of pregnancy and birth—unlike almost any other medical condition—isn't about simply avoiding risk. It's about creating a family. Ideally, there is room for both languages to be spoken and heard.

Having been the chair of an ob-gyn department, I'm all too aware that old practices can take too long to die out. Physicians, especially while committed to the scientific method, often bristle at changing their practice. Metrics, protocols, and outcomes data help, but so do humor, humility, and grace.

Pregnancy and childbirth can bring us indescribable joy—and sometimes extreme pain. Making new life is unavoidably messy and raw, but ideally, we emerge transformed in the best sense. There's no right way to have a child; it has always been a collaboration between patient, practitioner, family, and friends. I've been privileged to share in so many of those journeys, and I can confidently say that you're lucky to have Leslie Schrock along on yours.

Jane van Dis, MD, FACOG

PREFACE

I was pregnant for almost sixteen consecutive months before my first son arrived. The same time it takes to gestate a baby rhinoceros.

The first pregnancy ended early. I miscarried while traveling.

The second started just two weeks later. It was declared not viable at twelve weeks and ended in a medically necessary abortion.

The third pregnancy began after a two-month break. My son, the baby rhino, was pulled out of my belly wailing nine months later.

Those sixteen months taught me a lot.

I learned that it's possible to get pregnant almost every cycle you try, even if you are over thirty-five. That your body can take repeated hormonal punishment and stretching in strange places and still be strong. That even with optimism and preparation, birth, breastfeeding, and so many parts of the journey will not go as you plan. That knowledge, honesty, a sense of humor, and friends are essential at every turn. That growing a new human is only the first stage of metamorphosis to parent. And that there is so much about pregnancy that no one talks about.

After spending over a decade working in health, I came to pregnancy with more knowledge than most. So if it was this surprising for me, what was pregnancy like for everyone else? I went deep into the research, interviewed dozens of healthcare providers and complementary practitioners, and talked to new and experienced parents about what they wish they'd known. That research yielded the first edition of *Bumpin'*, which was written in real time during my pregnancy with the aforementioned baby rhino.

Since his arrival, there have been two more pregnancies. The first ended in another miscarriage; the second, a year later, resulted in a second healthy baby boy. Now, after five total pregnancies, this uterus is officially closed for business. While winding down my baby-making years, I researched and wrote a second book—*Fertility Rules*—to help everyone at the beginning of theirs. It's an evidence-backed guide to reproductive health that you can think of as a prequel to *Bumpin'*. Over the past five years, I have also fielded many questions from readers and friends (who now call me pregnancy Siri), continued conversations with medical experts and scientists, and read hundreds of journal articles to keep up with the ever-changing research landscape. The result of that analysis is this deeply revised second edition, which builds an even broader, more holistic view of family-building from conception through pregnancy and into the postpartum period.

So, what are you about to read? *Bumpin'* is a mix of science, practical advice, and a dash of personal experience. It combines the latest clinical research with guidance on topics like financial planning, exercise, what to buy (and what to skip), working while pregnant and after birth, and how to handle changing relationships with your partner and friends. It also helps you build more communicative, positive relationships with your providers and teaches you how to advocate for yourself in healthcare settings. And it doesn't skip the hard parts, like fertility issues, miscarriage, and changes during the postpartum period. Or real talk about topics like CBD and Botox. And the questions you may be too embarrassed to ask, like, Will sleeping on my stomach hurt the baby? (Nope!)

We'll cover all five of pregnancy's adventurous trimesters, so you're not left hanging if you run into questions during conception or after birth. Trimester zero is all about getting pregnant; trimesters one through three are the period spent baking your wee human; and the fourth trimester is the first three months postpartum. Each section starts with symptoms and solutions, advice for your partner, and a to-do list. Then we'll go deeper and tackle the major decisions and events you'll face at each stage.

My explicit goal is *not* to focus on things that are frequently out of your control, or to perpetuate the idea that every pregnancy and baby is the same. Just because something worked for your friend or sister doesn't mean it will for you. Happily, there are many tools to individualize your experience. Sections that cover finding different providers, evaluating prenatal testing, and debunking long-held myths in areas like exercise and food are written in that spirit. And instead of prescribing a specific path through pregnancy, there are trimester-by-trimester frameworks so you can decide what best meets your family's needs and preferences.

Maternal mortality rates, especially for women of color, are disgracefully high. And it doesn't have to be this way. Eighty percent of pregnancy-related deaths are preventable. You know your body best and should never be afraid to call your provider if something feels off. Our bodies are designed to create and gestate babies and give birth. Humans have done it billions of times. However, it has always been a miraculous, imperfect process, and encountering difficulty does not make you a failure, nor does it make you any less of a parent. The idea that any birth is unnatural is ridiculous, and as you'll read later, the history of the so-called natural childbirth movement is not what most people think. We'll also refer to pain medications and interventions as medicated or unmedicated, and birth types as vaginal or C-section.

If you're picking up this book because you want to understand what your partner or friend or surrogate is experiencing, good for you! There are plenty of ways to be helpful, and you'll learn about the big changes in store throughout the book. Later, you'll need to keep an eye on her health as she recovers, too.

If your partner hasn't picked up this book yet, give it to them when you're done. Even better: Start a book club and read together and discuss as you go.

Now, on to what's new in this second edition. There are updates to the data throughout that reflect the latest research across every area, from medical guidelines to miscarriage. There is a new chapter on exercise and nutrition, including simple things you can do at home to deal with aches and pains. The birth preferences (it's not a plan!) section has also been extended. The number one request I've received over the years—how to create a baby budget—is addressed here too. So are more personal stories that reflect the perspective I have as a now parent of two.

This second edition also goes far deeper into the postpartum period, as I find it strange that every other book stops at the moment you give birth. As if the experience stops there! The postpartum period is a surprise to nearly all first-time moms (also dads) and rarely (if ever) matches the polished version online, which is missing the context of the time, effort, resources, and retouching required to achieve snap-back abs (among other things). The internet can be a helpful place to turn for community depending on where you hang out, and there are many supportive pregnancy groups. But it is also a cesspool of mommy shaming, carried out by the last people you'd expect—other mothers. It's easy to have strong opinions, and pregnancy, birth, and parenting are (believe me) polarizing topics. But it's hard enough to be a parent today without having to fear public castigation. You never know what's happening in someone else's life: Lead with kindness and give your fellow preggos (and parents) a break.

One of my favorite new additions was born of my own experience, and that of so many struggling moms I've spoken to over the past several years. Breastfeeding seems like it should come naturally, but women are not born knowing how, and there is little lactation support unless you can pay for it. Sometimes it works and is magical, and other times it is relentless and hard. The world is not designed to support breastfeeding, and most mothers do not have the community, family, or financial support necessary to be with their babies all day, every day, exclusively breastfeeding for months. Companies rarely provide on-site day care or other resources for new mothers to breastfeed their babies at work—they offer pumping policies at best. While pumping allows women to keep up their milk supply, it does not allow for bonding time.

The systems that cause these structural failures are slow to change, so parents are left to manage the best they can and are often left feeling disappointed. Formula still gets a bad rap, but today's versions are far better than they used to be, with some recent additions to the market that seek to replicate the nutritional benefits of breast milk.

Trimester zero also got a big upgrade based on research from *Fertility Rules*. One in six people globally struggle with infertility, yet the emotional and societal burdens are shouldered almost entirely by women. But fun fact: Though men aren't tested or treated at the same rates as women, issues in their bodies cause around half of all infertility. Unlike eggs, which once abnormal cannot be fixed, sperm regenerate constantly, and men can improve their fertility often through simple lifestyle changes. With that in mind, there are new sections that explore what to do if you experience a miscarriage, run into fertility challenges, or undergo assisted reproduction treatments like IVF, and how infertility can affect you later as a parent. This includes current parents, as secondary infertility (the inability to get or stay pregnant after you've already welcomed one or more children) is more common than most people know.

Even though five years have passed since this book first came out, we still have a long way left to go with pregnancy research. The ethics of exposing pregnant women and babies to the risks of research in a gold-standard, randomly controlled trial is one reason many studies are done with animals, have low sample sizes, or rely on self-reported data. The other is that women are still underrepresented in clinical trials overall. In 1977, the FDA recommended excluding all women of reproductive age from research as a reaction to the drug thalidomide, a sedative used in Europe and Canada that caused horrific limb deformities in the children of the pregnant women who took it. It wasn't until 1993 that the NIH mandated women return to trials. Women's health research is also underfunded, so between the years we lost and money still required, there are not definitive answers to some questions you may have. New findings can also change the minds of the most august medical organizations, and studies are also sometimes proven incorrect or are found not to be repeatable, even by the scientists who performed the originals. In other words, if you're panic reading studies that pop up in the media, take it all with a very large grain of salt.

If you really can't help yourself, here are a few quick ways to evaluate whether a study is worth your attention. First, look at the sample size, which should be large and representative of the general population. Also take a look at who (or what organization) is funding the research and whether their sponsorship raises a conflict of interest for the research team. Academic researchers are under significant pressure by their institutions to publish papers, and the more interesting and unique their findings are, the more likely a journal editor is to bite. Confounding factors, the variables related to the supposed cause and supposed effect of a study, can be difficult to untangle too. Lastly, correlation is not causation. Many studies that land in your feeds do not meet all (or any) of the standards above. And there's one other thing: Clinical medicine is an average of seventeen years behind research. In other words, the study you read may not make it into your ob-gyn's or midwife's office in time for it to affect your pregnancy (though it never hurts to ask).

All research and clinical guidelines in this book have been evaluated by a team of medical experts and edited by my insightful, experienced ob-gyn partner, Jane van Dis, MD. Go to the bibliography for further reading. This book's practical side reflects hundreds of conversations and interviews with medical professionals and experts, from ob-gyns to reproductive endocrinologists and urologists, physical therapists, mental health providers, and pelvic floor therapists, and the collective wisdom of experienced parents who have been exactly where you are.

ONE LAST THING . . .

Starting a family is rarely a straightforward journey. Even if things are smooth, it's a long one, as the average pregnancy is 280 days, or 6,720 hours long. This is the first of many reminders that asking for help doesn't make you weak or incompetent. Childbearing and child-rearing have always taken a village, and there is no better time to prepare for that reality than before your tiny human shows up.

I hope this book leaves you empowered to face whatever this wild, weird, and wonderful journey throws your way, teaches you at least one fact worth repeating, and is as fun for you to read as it was for me to write.

Note: For those starting this journey as part of the LGBTQ+ communities, we standardize the pronouns she *and* her, *and refer to the birth parent as a woman and mother for purposes of simplicity to all readers.*

Trimester Zero

Welcome to the wild, sometimes painful, emotional, magical journey that is pregnancy. Whether you are just starting, it's your second or third time around, you're accompanying someone else, or pondering it for the future, deciding to conceive is the first of many life-altering moments to come. Your journey, like your eventual baby, will be unique to you, so lesson one is to try not to compare it to those of friends or families, or to stories you read online. Nature has an independent agenda, so even if you do everything "right," unfortunately no one is in full control of this process.

That said, there are plenty of choices you can control, and conception is the first opportunity to optimize your care, body, and life. Trimester Zero covers how to get your bodies and lives (that's right—yours and your partner's) ready, followed by a refresher on how making a baby works, in case your only formal training was during middle school sex ed. We'll also tackle what to do if you run into challenges (without letting them preemptively freak you out) and the wide range of solutions that exist to help you build a family today.

Greetings, friend! To separate the facts from the personal commentary, these italicized sections appear throughout to recount my journey from conception all the way through postpartum. If you're just here for the science, feel free to skip 'em. But if you decide to read on, I promise to be brutally honest.

GET READY

Preconception health, buying the perfect
prenatal vitamin, creating your first
baby budget, and preparing for parenting

I f you are already pregnant, congratulations, and keep reading; there is still plenty here for you. Pregnancy preparation is almost always focused on a woman's physical health and what to eat and do. While less discussed parts of the experience like quitting birth control (and its accompanying gnarly hormone changes) are important to understand, if your partner is providing sperm, they should commit to a cleanup, since their health impacts fertility, pregnancy, and future children too.

It's not just about the raw materials. Most new parents will tell you their relationship changed after having a baby. Some shift in wonderful ways, like feeling more bonded. Other changes are less great, like having limited time together (at least, sans baby), less frequent sex and intimacy, or experiencing feelings of bitterness tied to lopsided responsibilities. And how could such a major event *not* change things?

Family therapists suggest talking about your individual and shared parenting and life expectations early and often before the fog of pregnancy hormones descends. Topics can span the financial and personal implications of childcare, parental leave, sharing baby care and household duties, and values related to how you want to raise your child.

Why do this now? Resentment is a huge issue for many couples.

More women stay home to take care of their families than men, and almost all women, regardless of their professional status, take on more household responsibilities. Even in families where both partners work, moms do most scheduling and cleaning and are more likely to stay home when children get sick. In the early days with an infant, especially if you're breastfeeding, an equitable division of baby care is not a realistic goal—unless men can be biologically reprogrammed to lactate. But there are plenty of ways your partner can contribute (sanitation crew, anyone?).

Pregnancy is the wildest transformation of most women's lives. At times, you won't feel, look, or even act like yourself. And no matter how marvelous or tuned-in your partner is, they will not completely understand the physical and emotional undertaking that is growing another human. Instead of expecting psychic powers to miraculously appear, tell them directly how to best support you, and be honest about how you're feeling. Ask them the same questions. They aren't living with the day-to-day of pregnancy, but this is a seismic transition for them, too.

FOR PARTNERS

Speaking of partners, hello, you! Hopefully you're reading the whole book, but for those skimming, these sections are packed with the advice experienced parents wish they'd known. Before our first chat, let's say the quiet part out loud: Your role (and you) will often feel secondary. But there are plenty of ways to get involved before, during, and after pregnancy. Think of these callouts as cheat codes to anticipate and sidestep the common issues couples encounter and keep your relationship healthy. Starting now.

Take your lifestyle and health seriously

Women's bodies and choices are blamed first if conception is a struggle—not, if you are a heterosexual male, on you. Ironically, around half of all fertility issues are related to sperm and men's bodies (one-third are exclusively related to women, one-third to men, and one-third are a combination or unknown). Given that you are contributing half of your child's genetic material, what you do matters, too. Eating a diet packed with whole, unprocessed foods (especially avoiding added sugars and trans fats), staying active, moderating alcohol consumption, and avoiding sperm killers like saunas, cycling, smoking, THC and other recreational drugs, and steroids is a great place to start. No need to load up on supplements unless you have a deficiency—a high-quality multivitamin or a prenatal formulated for men is plenty.

Be patient and keep things light

Conception can quickly become a stressful and obsessive process, especially timing sex during fertile windows. Add hormonal changes (if a woman just quit taking birth control) or worry when things don't happen immediately, and any joy in the creation of new life can vanish.

Your mission, should you choose to accept it: Be patient, find ways to defuse the anxiety, and keep life fun. Schedule a date night. Keep each other distracted, especially if getting pregnant takes longer than you'd like. Communicate openly, and even if you're not the type to talk about your feelings, be honest about how you are dealing.

BOOK A PRECONCEPTION CHECKUP

If you already have a physician in mind to manage your prenatal care, now is a great time to schedule a chat about improving your fertility and how to have a healthy pregnancy. Not sure? Set an appointment with your ob-gyn or gynecologist. Yes, partners, this advice is for you, too. Some prescription drugs impact sperm quality and quantity, so ideally, book an appointment at least three months before you start trying to conceive (TTC) so you can adjust if needed.

When you go in for an appointment, prepare for a slew of questions that will determine whether your pregnancy will require anything beyond standard-issue prenatal care, or extra steps during conception. Partners, you'll hear many of the same questions, especially related to lifestyle, family history, and genetic screenings.

Here are the topics you can expect to discuss:

- Age
- Family history
- Gynecological history (state of your menstrual cycle, current or past methods of birth control, STDs or abnormal Pap smears, history of infertility or past pregnancies)
- Medical history (preexisting conditions, past surgeries or hospitalizations, exposure to infectious diseases)
- Medications and allergies (all prescription or OTC medications and supplements, including prenatal vitamins, and known allergies)
- Vaccinations (childhood history, Tdap [tetanus, diphtheria, acellular pertussis], flu shot, and upcoming travel requiring vaccines)
- Lifestyle (profession; hobbies; relationship status; use of drugs, alcohol, tobacco, and caffeine; exercise, weight and dietary history)
- Emotional history (history of anxiety, depression or mood disorders, eating disorders, current or past domestic violence or sexual assault/rape)
- Genetic carrier screening (family history of birth defects, abnormalities, inherited disorders, miscarriage, or stillbirth)

Depending on the answers, your physician may order tests, get you up-to-date with missing vaccines, and make lifestyle-related suggestions. While it's tempting to downplay questionable behavior with your physician, now is not the time for half-truths. One common example: Studies show that women often conceal how much alcohol they consume. If your practitioner is given incomplete or slightly fudged information, they can't provide the best care. So both of you: Please tell the truth.

Now back to you, ladies. Let's get real: Pregnancy is a weird time for your body. New medical problems can start, ongoing issues can get worse, and all these changes can affect the safety and efficacy of medications you've taken for years. If you have a chronic condition, or take anything to manage your health, it's important to chat with your prescribing physician before trying to conceive. It's not always a straightforward decision to stay on, make a change to, or get off some prescriptions entirely, and balancing the trade-offs is best done in partnership with your provider. You may already know where to start since most drugs are labeled with reproductive health warnings for pregnant and lactating women. Regarding male fertility and reproductive health? Not so much, which is why it's so important for partners to do a workup too.

FERTILITY TESTING

If you want more insight into your reproductive health, there are a growing number of direct-to-consumer fertility tests on the market. If you're fertility curious, this is the best route, as doing the same panel in-office with your doctor without an underlying problem will not be covered by insurance. That said, if an abnormal result comes back, your doctor will rerun the test again in their own lab.

At-home hormone tests are usually done via blood spot, which involves pricking your finger with a lancet and filling tiny circles on a card with blood, then mailing it back. For women, the markers they test are related to ovarian reserves (the number of available eggs in your ovaries) as well as ovulation and testosterone. For men, testosterone, estradiol, dehydroepiandrosterone (DHEA), and cortisol are the key markers tested. To evaluate sperm, the process is similar, though it requires a different sort of contribution and immediate drop-off for overnight delivery at your favorite shipping service. The test results are emailed, or released during another phone consultation with a physician, who will walk you through the findings.

Testing isn't mandatory, but if you have irregular cycles or reason to believe that you may have an underlying gynecological condition like PCOS (polycystic ovary syndrome) or endometriosis, talk about it in your preconception appointment and see if your provider thinks it's necessary. In-clinic testing is done via traditional blood draws in your doctor's lab of choice.

GENETIC CARRIER SCREENINGS

A genetic carrier screening reveals whether you or your partner carry genetic markers for any of several health conditions, and how likely it is that your child will inherit it. Done via blood draw, saliva sample, or cheek swab, it's noninvasive and tests primarily for cystic fibrosis, sickle cell disease, fragile X syndrome, and Tay-Sachs disease. Direct-to-consumer tests are available, but if you think you might be at higher risk, it's best to do this screening through your physician. Why do it? Some conditions don't present in every generation, so you may not know about them. Also, recalling the medical histories of every single family member is challenging enough, even if you have decent records.

Just in case you slept through high school biology, here is a crash course on genetic inheritance. After cultivating and testing thousands of pea plants, a monk named Gregor Mendel discovered that several basic principles applied to the passing of traits from parents to their offspring. These basic principles are known as Mendel's laws and go like this: Offspring inherit one genetic marker from each parent independent of any others, and recessive markers will always be masked by those that are dominant.

Screenings start with a full medical history, and the partner with a higher carrier risk will be tested first. The types of conditions your doctor may ask about are more varied, and you may not be as susceptible to some based on your background. If the results from the first partner's round of testing are clean, there is no need to do another, as it takes both of you for a condition to be an issue.

If you are both carriers for a serious condition, there are options. You can choose to get pregnant and rely on diagnostic tests to confirm whether your baby inherited the condition. IVF using your own sperm and eggs or donor gametes is another option. The fertilized embryos can be tested before implantation to ensure you will not pass the condition down. A genetic counselor or physician will guide this process, so you won't be making these decisions alone.

AU REVOIR TO BIRTH CONTROL

Hormonal birth control works (for the most part) by stopping ovulation; no ovulation, no pregnancy. So if you're taking birth control or have an IUD, the first big step in downshifting to conception mode is to stop or take it out. If you're on the pill, you can quit whenever you want, though your bleeding schedule and ovulation may be irregular.

When does normal fertility return? The answer: much more quickly than you might think. With most hormonal forms, including the pill and IUD, there is only a transient delay of a few weeks or months, and in some cases, ovulation and a normal cycle come back immediately. Same with the copper IUD, which contains zero hormones and does not impact ovulation (sperm really hate copper). The birth control shot is the only form with a longer timeline, of up to nine months.

For long-term users, stopping hormonal birth control can be a BIG transition, so expect some hormonal and mood changes. Gone too will be the days of a light, predictable, symptom-free flow, if you were lucky enough to experience that. But good news: If birth control knocked down your libido, it may return once you stop.

Side effects of stopping birth control

- Heavier periods
- Cramps
- Irregular cycle length
- Acne
- Weight fluctuations
- Fewer headaches

GETTING TO KNOW YOUR CYCLE

If your period is regular and you were not on hormonal birth control, you may already have a record of your cycle. For those who haven't had one in a while or are putting birth control on the shelf, exactly when a period will return in full force is different for everyone. Some come right back the first month after stopping. Others take longer. Once it does make an appearance, it's best to complete at least one full cycle before trying to conceive, to pinpoint your fertile window more accurately. It also helps with more exact dating if you do get pregnant, as due dates are calculated based on the start of your last menstrual period (LMP).

Data points like your cycle length and blood volume and color in combination with a presence or lack of symptoms say a lot about the state of your fertility. We are all conditioned to think they are normal, but PMS symptoms like bloating, cramps, and acne can be signs of hormonal imbalances. If yours are extreme, talk to your favorite medical practitioner to debug.

Since you may be getting to know each other again, here are the basics of a normal, healthy menstrual cycle:

- **Cycle length:** twenty-five to thirty-five days (a consistent duration month to month is more important than length)
- **Bleeding duration:** four to seven days
- **Color:** bright red (think cranberry juice) with no clots

- **Volume:** Enough to fill up a tampon, pad, or cup in under four hours. If it's more than that for several cycles in a row, chat with your provider.

There are apps to track your period over time, or you can just mark it on a calendar. If you do choose to use an app, read their terms of service and privacy policy to ensure your data remains private and anonymous. If your period is irregular or otherwise out of whack, look to diet and lifestyle for simple tweaks. Stress, nutrition, exercise, and sleep all impact your menstrual cycle, so try drinking more water and less caffeine and alcohol to start. It's normal to spot during ovulation, but if you have breakthrough bleeding outside of that time, take note.

I was on the pill for almost twenty years to control cramping and digestive issues that started when I was a teenager. I barely had a trace of a period after I started taking it. Most months, it didn't even occur to me that I had a period, since bleeding was so rare. When I quit, I expected my cycle to take a while to return but was pleasantly surprised that it came back exactly twenty-eight days later.

My mood swings were a less pleasant surprise. Small things that normally didn't bother me, like dirty dishes in the sink, were all of a sudden a REALLY big deal. I was less touchy during pregnancy than in that first month off the pill.

We never expected to get pregnant the first time we tried, and on every subsequent attempt. Our semi-crazy fertility hit rate is not typical, but is one reason I advocate for prepping your body in advance, since pregnancy can happen before you expect it.

CHOOSING PRENATAL VITAMINS AND SUPPLEMENTS

Eating a well-rounded, veggie-packed diet during pregnancy can be tough, especially if first-trimester morning sickness ensures that all you can choke down is carbs. Combined with its proven reduction in neural tube and heart defects, preterm birth, low birth weights, and even autism, the magical prenatal vitamin, powered by folic acid, is key from conception through breastfeeding. All supplements beyond prenatals should be disclosed to and coordinated with your medical provider, as some are not pregnancy-safe (like vitamin A) or can interact with other medications.

When you go shopping, here are the ingredients to seek out on the label:

Vitamin	What is it and what is the benefit?
Folic acid (600–800 mcg is optimal)	A synthetic form of folate, or Vitamin B9; helps prevent neural tube defects and possibly other birth defects including cleft lip and palate.
Iron (27 mg)	A mineral that supports the development of the placenta and fetus and helps your body to make blood. It also helps prevent anemia, which can be more common during pregnancy.
Vitamin D (15 mcg; more if you have a deficiency)	Helps support the development of your baby's teeth and bones. Your vitamin D levels may be tested if you're at risk for low levels. Look for D3 on the label, as it's more readily converted into vitamin D's active form and raises blood concentrations for longer.

Iodine (220 mcg)	A trace element important to fetal neurodevelopment.
Omega-3 fatty acids (200–300 mg)	These support fetal brain and eye development and immune function. DHA and EPA will come in some prenatal supplement bundles but cannot be packaged in tablets, as they are oils.
Choline (450 mg)	A nutrient that is important to fetal brain and spine development. It's not found in all prenatal formulations, so take it as an extra supplement if necessary, or if yours doesn't have a high enough dose, as few do.

It is not always possible to get the optimal NRV (nutrient reference value) in a single capsule or pill, and some formulations are strong across most areas but do not contain omega-3 fatty acids (DHA and EPA) or enough of other ingredients like calcium and magnesium. If you think you need to supplement further, talk to your provider about your diet and see what they suggest. Prenatal vitamin side effects are usually minimal, but the iron can cause constipation and nausea, so take them at night before you go to bed, with a snack, or look for food-based versions that are easier to digest.

Partners, there are two options for you: a high-quality multivitamin, or a male prenatal vitamin. The latter will be formulated with CoQ10; vitamins C, D, and E; folate; lycopene; selenium; and zinc, which are all critical to sperm health. For most men, multivitamins are also just fine.

Selecting high-quality supplements

Before you start taking any supplements beyond a prenatal, have a chat with your ob-gyn or midwife. The human body does its most effective absorption of vitamins and minerals through food, so the goal is to eat a well-rounded diet and only supplement as needed beyond a prenatal. Supplements in the US are regulated like food, not drugs, even though they can have pharmaceutical-grade effects in the body. So even though they are now often packaged as gummies, they are not candy.

On that note, many gummy prenatals do not contain iron or, due to the process required to manufacture them, enough of the ingredients above to be effective. Gummy vitamins are a sugar-packed, inferior method of vitamin and mineral delivery versus tablets and softgels, so choose another form unless you have no other option. Softgels can contain DHA and EPA, and often come packaged together with a tablet for brands that provide an all-in-one bundled solution. No matter what supplement you're selecting, here are the rules to live by:

- Choose a company that lists information about their supply chain and traceability, and that performs third-party testing. This means an outside organization has tested and certified the nutritional values and contents of the product. Ask for a certificate of analysis (COA) if you want proof.
- Expensive doesn't always mean better—sometimes you're paying for growth marketing, not high-quality ingredients.
- Beware of bona fides and recommendations by influencers and doctors—these are paid ads.
- "Natural" means nothing on a supplement label; checking sourcing practices is a more effective way to know what's going into your body.
- Look below the label at the list of ingredients. If there is a paragraph of words you don't understand, those are synthetic fillers, and that formulation should be avoided.

CREATING A BABY BUDGET

Getting a handle on your health and conceiving is only part of the having-a-kid equation. The other major but less acknowledged component? Money.

It may seem premature to talk about baby budgets before you are pregnant. But raising a child from birth to age seventeen costs over $300,000 for middle-income families, and the first year alone can run over $20,000. These numbers do not include a college education, nor do they account for indirect costs like your time, lost earnings, or missed career opportunities. In the first years of life, the biggest financial outlays are for childcare, gear like diapers and formula, and medical expenses. Exact expenses vary depending on where you live, but the high costs of these goods and services, especially childcare, come as a surprise to three of every four new parents. Three-quarters of expectant parents assume childcare costs won't impact their career decisions, but 63 percent report later that they did.

The surprise costs of having children can also have unsavory effects on a couple's emotional well-being. A study spanning thirty-five countries, eight years, and over a million people showed that having kids lowered happiness until you controlled for the ability to pay your bills. For couples who plan for these costs, building a family is more likely to be a positive. Exactly how you divide and manage financial responsibilities is unique to your careers, your relationship dynamic, long-term goals, and how you visualize the first few years of your child's life. The earlier you plan and talk about this together, the more prepared you will be to handle surprises, and the less likely you are to fight later.

To start a baby budget, look at your current finances, available savings, income, and existing monthly burn rate, or the amount that goes out the door. You can set a baseline goal using the 50/30/20 rule, meaning you allocate 50 percent of income into needs like food, rent, or a mortgage; 30 percent for wants like that chic Scandinavian changing table; and 20 percent to pay off debt or put into savings. Many families need more than a 50 percent allocation for essentials, so adjust as needed and remember that the whole point is to track and make goals and get rid of financial obstacles that keep you from focusing on other priorities. If either of you is planning to take unpaid leave or stop working, you may want to practice living on less before you have to.

When it comes to the baby, there will be large up-front costs, like medical expenses and stocking a nursery, and smaller recurring costs, like childcare and diapers. A review of your health plan will tell you if your desired birth spot, complementary practitioners, and pre/post services (if you have already chosen these things) are covered. But even if your coverage is excellent, it's best to set aside an emergency medical fund for the unexpected.

A standard health plan generally covers:
- Pre- and postnatal doctor's appointments, labs, medications, and treatments or screenings for conditions like gestational diabetes
- Inpatient experiences including birth, hospitalizations, and assorted hospital fees
- Breast pump and lactation counseling
- Newborn care (shots and tests done in the hospital, vaccines, well-baby visits)

Pro tip: Pregnancy is not a "qualifying life event" that allows you to change your insurance coverage outside of open enrollment periods—but birth is. In the thirty to sixty days after the baby pops out, you can add Junior and make further changes to your plan. Upgrading or downgrading afterward will not affect costs related to birth. However, if you decided to go premium while pregnant and want to move to a less expensive plan when you're done, it's possible. Just consider the five to seven pediatrician appointments in your baby's first year of life before you cut, as costs for vaccinations and those visits add up.

One other thing: Pregnancy is a perfect time to spend those stored FSA (flexible spending account) or HSA (health savings account) dollars.

If these accounts are new concepts, think of them as savings accounts built with pretax dollars funneled directly from your paycheck. Spend them on copays, deductibles, prenatal vitamins, baby-related medical items, or postpartum items for yourself. If you run out of ideas, stock up on sunscreen.

We'll dive into the pros and cons of different childcare options later, but ask yourself early (and honestly) what kind of help you need and on what timeline. The answer will reflect how much parental leave each of you receive, when (and whether) you plan to return to work, your budget, and your desires as a parent. If you will rely on family for childcare, it's crucial to set expectations early (and often) so you know you have a reliable baseline and can communicate about what's working and what's not. If day care is the plan, lists can fill up far in advance, so it's best to investigate before you're pregnant or during the first trimester. Nannies and nanny shares are more expensive options that provide more flexibility and support, and finding the right fit usually takes four to six weeks. Apart from day care, you'll need to identify backup options in the event of illness or unforeseen events, too.

Most parents who stock up on clothes, toys, and gadgets before getting to know their baby's preferences will tell you they should have waited. Humans successfully raised children for thousands of years before BabyBjörn. So, while outfitting a nursery and accessorizing your baby is fun, you can minimize costs by renting equipment you'll only use for a short period of time (like bassinets), borrowing from friends and family, and buying secondhand from one of the many online marketplaces or mom groups. The biggest ongoing infant expenses you can't avoid are diapers and, if you aren't breastfeeding, formula (though breastfeeding isn't free either—we'll cover that later). You'll wear maternity clothes for only a few months, so look in your closet for pieces with extra room or that will stretch to accommodate your growing belly, borrow, buy used, or rent before investing in a spendy pregnancy wardrobe. If you're planning for future children, consider buying some gender-neutral pieces so you can reuse everything later.

To understand baseline costs during pregnancy and the first three months postpartum, here is a template with general categories and a list of items you'll need from pregnancy through the first year with an infant. Use this to do product research; decide what's going on the baby registry, as friends and family will absolutely want to buy you fun, less essential things; and start a discussion with your partner. These costs change based on geography, what kind of employee benefits or insurance you have, and which specific items you choose to buy.

Category	Items
Healthcare expenses	Copays/screenings, birth, well-baby visits, baby vaccinations/boosters, postpartum support, and out-of-pocket expenses like a doula
Recurring costs	Baby supplies including diapers; wipes; formula; laundry detergent; lotion; shampoo and wash; new, age-appropriate toys and books; clothes
Childcare	Day care, in-home care, nanny share, nanny, etc.
Onetime baby purchases	See baby registry section for a full list but should include items like furniture, bouncer, changing pad, burp cloths, baby bathtub, grooming kit, infant thermometer, crib and/or pack 'n' play, crib sheets and mattress, infant car seat, stroller, play mat, nasal aspirator, monitor, diaper pail, and bibs.
Mom purchases	Prenatal vitamins (starting at least three months before TTC [trying to conceive] through breastfeeding), pumping and nursing bras, maternity clothes, breastfeeding pillow, birth recovery kit (postpartum underwear and/or pads, sitz bath, etc.)

The mind reels that there could be more to say about money in this book. But there is an important financial concept that matters even in year one of a child's life: compound interest. You can give your kids a head start by financially utilizing the magic of compound interest, which adds up significantly over time. Start by setting up a high-yield savings account or individual retirement account (IRA) and contributing whatever you can afford each month after your baby is born. By the time your baby hits eighteen, the money you tucked away each year will have grown into a meaningful amount that can be used for college or anything else your child needs.

PARENTING GOALS

We assume everyone building a family is ready for it. Here's a secret: Even the most relaxed, assured-looking parents who plan for years have moments, especially when they're sleep deprived and faced with an inconsolable newborn at 3:00 a.m. Parenting has many seasons, from the pre-kid life you'll have trouble remembering during those bleary infant days and eventually a kid who thinks he's fourteen even though he's four.

A big mental hurdle for most first-time mothers and fathers is deciding how they want to show up in the world as parents. This identity is tied to so many things—age, professional experience, how you perceive gender roles and responsibilities, your own childhood, and financial resources, to name a few. Everyone also enters parenting as someone else's child. We learn habits and behaviors from our parents, which affect the way we approach our own roles as parents. Your upbringing does not dictate who you become but can have unintended side effects if you don't take the time to process it. Whether your childhood was complicated or great or somewhere in between, try to reflect on who your parents are, why they did what they did, and how it affected you. Kudos if you've already covered this in therapy. If it's still difficult, it may be worth recruiting professional help.

If you'd like to explore your parenting identity and practice co-parenting communication, start by asking yourself why you want to have a child, and if you have a specific idea of what your future family will look like. There is no right answer, just what feels right to you. Then consider what kind of parent you'd like to be. Share with your significant other and see how their personal vision overlaps with yours. Even if you've talked about it before, you might find there are areas where you diverge now that it's all becoming real. Take a few minutes several times a week to check in with each other. Talk about your days, about what's working at home, what's not, and what needs to change. If you're not always face-to-face, this can also happen asynchronously via text, voice, or video message. If you wait to form these habits until an infant is around, they probably won't stick. As time goes on, these conversations will evolve, as will your individual and shared identities.

When your new addition does finally make his or her appearance, keep the lines of communication open and share your parenting philosophy with others, especially caregivers, family, and friends. If you have a specific value system or set of principles, it's important to be surrounded by others who share (or are at least willing to adhere to) them.

Figuring out what doesn't work is just as important as discovering what does, and effort goes a long way even when you make mistakes. And you will make mistakes—every parent does. Kids have a baseline that you can't always control, and your relationship with them shouldn't always be about discipline. We listen to people we trust, so through conversation, consistency, and flexibility, you can help your children trust you.

MAKING A BABY

Eggs, sperm, ovulation, sex,
the two-week wait, and taking THE TEST

Though it probably seems like some couples just look at each other and *bam!* are pregnant, that is not the case for everyone. You may already know the basics of when and how you can get pregnant from sex ed, your parents, friends, or your favorite fertility app. But no matter what you think you know, it's important to calibrate your expectations.

I know what you're thinking: You are one of those people who got pregnant every time you tried. Yes, it's true, but our conception hit rate was unusual. That said, I followed all the advice below: I learned to understand the ebbs and flows of my cycle, tracked ovulation, and had sex on the optimal days (but not five times per day!). I also found ways to unwind and distract myself, mostly through exercise, acupuncture, and long walks with friends. My husband, Nick, made the same lifestyle improvements—more sleep, better diet, and moderate exercise—before we started trying too.

THE TRUTH ABOUT AGE AND FERTILITY

Fact: The day you turn thirty-five, your eggs do not shrivel up, nor do your odds of getting pregnant go to zero. In fact, there is a dramatic rise in the number of women who wait to have their first child. Since the 1970s, the number of first-time births to mothers thirty-five or older has increased ninefold. The practice of defining "advanced maternal age" as thirty-five or older is decades old and, just like the term itself, long overdue for an update.

Here's the truth. You are born with between one and two million eggs. By your first period, your supply drops to three hundred thousand. Though you'll ovulate only about four hundred times in your life, each month you'll lose around one thousand potential eggs. But the number of eggs you have does not dictate your ability to get pregnant. In fact, a low ovarian reserve (AMH [anti-Mullerian hormone] level on a hormone test) is not a good single indicator of your overall fertility.

What is true after thirty-five is that egg quality goes down, and your odds of having an embryo with a chromosomal abnormality increase. This is the main cause of higher miscarriage rates and of the rising chance that your child will have a condition like Down syndrome. One in 100 women are affected by premature ovarian failure (loss of normal ovarian function) before age forty. If you have a family history, talk to your doctor.

During your early twenties, 90 percent of all eggs are normal, and couples have a 96 percent chance of conceiving in under a year. From your fertile peak between twenty-four and thirty-four, your odds go to 86 percent after a year. At thirty, your conception success rate is still high—78 percent through age thirty-nine. At forty, female fertility gets a little more complicated. Your odds of getting pregnant each month drop to 5 percent. It's still possible to have a healthy pregnancy, as the limiting factor is typically egg quality, not the ability to successfully carry a pregnancy. But you might require assistance.

It's also true that men experience age-related fertility decline. Degrading sperm causes men's fertility rate to drop by half between thirty and forty, and though it's not as steep as women's, there is a significant drop at forty for men, too. Sperm quality is falling globally for reasons unknown, but we assume at least some is due to endocrine disruption and lifestyle. Since men regenerate sperm constantly, many issues can be improved with simple adjustments, so ensure your partner is doing the same healthy things you are.

HOW OVULATION WORKS

It's been a while since you got "the talk" after your first period arrived. Those that lived through that cringey conversation may remember that its primary focus was about how *not* to get pregnant rather than biology and fertile windows. Boys don't get much information on any of these topics, so read on for a refresher or, in many cases, a first education.

A textbook menstrual cycle is between twenty-four and thirty-eight days long. Its purpose: to prepare the human body for pregnancy. At the beginning of each cycle, estrogen and progesterone mature an egg in one of your ovaries and make the lining of your uterus thick and spongy. Halfway through, your right or left ovary (usually they alternate months) releases this mature egg through one of your fallopian tubes into the uterus in a process called ovulation. If the egg is fertilized by sperm, it burrows into the newly inviting uterine lining and begins a pregnancy. If it isn't fertilized, the lining breaks down and the resulting blood and tissue flow out as your period.

When you're ready to get pregnant on purpose, your focus is on the fertile window before the middle of the cycle—three days before and up to the day of ovulation. The fertile window is the most likely time you will successfully become pregnant, as the egg is available to be fertilized for only twelve to twenty-four hours. Sperm, on the other hand, can hang out and live in the reproductive organs for as long as five days, which is why having sex *before* you ovulate is a more successful route. It's also a leading cause of the around half of pregnancies that are not intended.

So how do you know if you're ovulating? Since every woman's cycle is slightly different, you have to pay attention. There are tried-and-true technology-free methods. And if you want to take things to the next level, you can pair them with one of the many apps and devices available to help you to see trends and, given time, predict when you'll ovulate based on your cycle's history.

Cervical mucus method

Cervical mucus is exactly what it sounds like—mucus that comes out of your cervix as vaginal discharge.

The same hormones that control the menstrual cycle—progesterone and estrogen—also influence the texture and appearance of cervical mucus. Right after your period, it will be light or possibly absent. As the egg matures, mucus increases in the vagina and will gradually get less cloudy. Cervical mucus around ovulation is clear and slippery, sometimes even stretchy, and resembles an egg white. This consistency is your sign that ovulation is under way.

If you want to give this method a whirl, get into a comfortable position, and reach one clean finger (index or middle is best) into your vagina and up toward your cervix to take a sample. Look at it and feel the consistency. If there isn't much going on or the mucus is sticky or creamy, it's not quite time. If it's slightly stretchy or wet, ovulation is near. If you get the holy grail of cervical mucus, stretchy egg whites, grab your partner—it's baby-making time. You can also check your underwear or toilet paper if you are in a rush. However, it may be harder to correctly assess what is going on.

Tip: Though many practitioners and women swear by it, this method is not always reliable or easy to interpret. It's especially difficult for those with sexually transmitted diseases, bacterial vaginosis or yeast infections, PCOS, or previous cervical surgeries, and for users of feminine hygiene products like douches or anything labeled as vaginal deodorant (please don't use them!). Cervical mucus monitoring must be done daily, especially during the period around and during your fertile window.

Basal body temperature method

This method demands the same daily diligence as cervical mucus monitoring. Your basal body temperature (BBT) is the temperature of your body at rest. To put together an accurate BBT chart, you'll need to take and record your temperature every morning as soon as you wake up and before you get out of bed. No bathroom breaks; you have to do it before you stand up. All you need is a basal body thermometer, which can be found at any drugstore for $10. They take slightly longer to give a result than the instant fever-detecting variety, as an accurate reading to the tenth of a degree makes all the difference.

So what do BBT readings tell you, exactly? During ovulation, your basal body temperature rises slightly from its normal state, by between 0.4 and 0.8° degrees Fahrenheit. The reading won't tell you precisely when the egg is released, but almost all women will ovulate within three days of that spike. BBT will stay at that spiked level until your period starts, then drop down again until the next cycle begins.

Tip: Many people also swear by BBT charting, but factors like sleep quality, having a fever, drinking or smoking the night before, or even going to the bathroom before measuring can throw off its accuracy. BBT needs to be measured at the same time every day to be correct.

The pee-on-a-stick method

Ovulation predictor kits (OPKs) detect the surge in luteinizing hormone (LH) twelve to thirty-six hours before you ovulate. This surge can last just hours, or as long as one to two days. Though there are tests that can be done with saliva or sweat, the most popular fluid input is urine. OPKs can be low-tech color-changing paper strips, or more advanced digital readers with smiley faces and pop-out test sticks, or even fertility monitors that you use all month long.

Each brand has slightly different requirements, so check the directions. The best practice is to test with first-thing-in-the-morning pee, and then again in the afternoon. Drinking too many fluids will dilute the results, so go easy on the liquids before you test.

Tip: Most ovulation tests detect that you are *about to* ovulate, but they can't confirm that you actually did unless they also test progesterone levels. Tests that detect progesterone are available but are more expensive. Women with irregular cycles or other menstrual issues like PCOS may have difficulty knowing when (and if) they ovulate. If you don't get a positive result during a cycle, it could mean one of several things. If you have a long cycle, you could be testing too soon. If you tested only in the morning, your LH surge might be short and not detectable until the afternoon. You also may not have ovulated that cycle or could be using a faulty test. This can happen with any brand, but is more common with cheap, bulk-packaged strips.

OPKs are great training wheels while you're learning the ropes of cervical mucus or BBT monitoring, and combined can paint a more complete picture of your fertility.

Fertility sensors

Into that passively-track-everything life? There are an increasing number of sensors and devices designed to make fertility tracking more frictionless by tracking physiological data and syncing it automatically with an app. Using parameters like skin temperature, resting pulse, heart rate variability, and sleep, they create a score that provides insight into your cycle and other indicators that can help you conceive.

Sensor designs can vary, from connected basal body thermometers to a vaginal sensor that measures your core body temperature, and bracelets and rings that track multiple parameters like resting pulse rate, stress, and movement while you sleep.

Tip: Before dropping hundreds of dollars, check the device's clinical trial data, which should be available on its website. Also be sure that your health profile fits the device's patient criteria, as many devices do not work well with fertility-related health conditions.

I tried all these methods and leaned most heavily on OPKs and an app that took historical cycle data to predict my ovulation date. Cervical mucus monitoring was not for me, as I had a hard time discerning the different consistencies. And even after leaving a BBT thermometer on my bedside table by my phone, inevitably I'd forget and get up to use the loo before using it.

DOING IT

Sex while trying to conceive isn't always *Kama Sutra*–level romantic, especially if you've been at it awhile or are attempting to time it with an ovulation peak. If you're not careful, it can start to feel like a job. So in the spirit of keeping this process as stress-free as possible, here are the answers to the most common sex-during-conception questions.

How many times do we need to have sex to conceive?

More is not always better. When men ejaculate too frequently, sperm quality and quantity goes down. When it doesn't happen enough, sperm can be too old and slow to get to the egg in a timely fashion. So though it seems logical to have sex five times per day during your fertile window, that is not the best way to get pregnant.

To optimize for sperm quality and getting them to their destination on time, have sex every other day or once per day *at most* in the five

days leading up to ovulation and on the day of. It is especially important not to overdo it if your partner has low-quality semen parameters.
Make sure your partner finishes ejaculating fully inside of you each
time.

What are the best positions?

Clinical research into pregnancy-friendly sexual positions is pretty
much nonexistent, and no one position has ever been proven more
effective than others. The two most recommended positions are
missionary and doggy style. They allow for deep penetration, and
in the case of missionary, the sperm is deposited directly into the
top of the vagina closer to the cervix. There are many variations,
like putting a pillow under your lower back in missionary to tilt
your hips up or lowering down flat from all fours in doggy style.
Rather than obsess about form and technique, mix things up and
have fun.

Will staying on my back afterward help?

The meeting of sperm and egg happens faster than you might think.
The entrance to the uterine canal is only a few centimeters long, and
in simulated studies, strong sperm travel at a rate of five millimeters
per minute, completing the whole journey from ejaculation to egg
in about ten minutes. They encounter barriers along the way that
are designed to filter out low-quality swimmers, like cervical mucus
and the vagina's acidic environment. Once the strong sperm make it
through the first round of the vaginal obstacle course into the uterus,
muscular contractions can help speed things up. Don't be concerned
about fluids that leak out afterward. Less than 5 percent of ejaculate
contains sperm.

There is no research showing whether a sideways postcoital snug-
gle or staying on your back after sex helps, nor is there proof that getting up immediately afterward hurts your chances. One reason people

believe they should stay on their backs with their feet on the wall is that fertility doctors often have intrauterine insemination (IUI) patients do it, even though there is no high-quality evidence that gravity makes a difference.

Anything else that can help my odds?

Avoid douching after sex and choose your lubricants wisely. If you need a little extra help, ensure your lube is fertility-friendly and does not contain spermicide or glycerin, which impedes and kills sperm. Water-based and pH balanced are two lubricant features to seek out, or there are specific products made especially for conception. Don't raise your core body temperature afterward with saunas, steam rooms, hot baths, or intense exercise, either, as those are all sperm killers.

The don't-make-it-a-job advice isn't just so you and your partner continue to have fun together. Too much stress can lower your chance of getting pregnant, so find ways to relax, and try not to obsess.

If you find yourself feeling less than enthused about more timed sex, as so many of us do, some couples turn to at-home kits for intra-vaginal or intracervical insemination (IVI and ICI). Akin to the turkey-baster method (but featuring FDA-cleared devices), this process allows a bit more flexibility around timing and releases the pressure of performing sexually on command.

THE WAIT, OR (WHAT FEELS LIKE) THE LONGEST TWO WEEKS OF YOUR LIFE

You've done the deed, you're hoping for the best, and now you must wait the fourteen or so days before your missed period. Rather than looking for early pregnancy symptoms before that missed period, for your own sanity seek out distractions and try not to think about it too much. Easier said than done, I know.

Early signs you might be pregnant

The most obvious is a missed period. But if you're on the lookout before it's due to arrive, there are other signs. Many of the symptoms below could be mistaken for PMS. It is tricky to know the difference, so rather than reading into every single small change, focus on taking good care of yourself until that missed period happens and you can test.

- Sensitive nipples
- Cramping
- Fatigue
- Nausea
- Frequent peeing (especially at night)
- Change in tastes and smells
- Moodiness
- Implantation bleeding

Implantation bleeding is especially confusing. It may seem counterintuitive, but around one-third of women experience spotting around the time the embryo implants in the uterine lining. Here are a few ways to differentiate implantation bleeding from your period:

- **Timing:** Typically happens a few days before your period is due, around ten days after you ovulated
- **Duration:** It can last for just hours or one to two days
- **Color:** Lighter pink or brownish in color versus the more vibrant cranberry color that marks your period
- **Cramping:** More mild cramping than your period, and no growing intensity

TAKING THE TEST

There are many types of pregnancy tests—digital, strips, compostable, those that involve smiley faces, paper, plastic—the list goes on. Though you may want to trust only the more expensive top-shelf tests with features like digital readouts, the underlying technology for detecting human chorionic gonadotropin (hCG), the hormone that placental cells produce during pregnancy, is the same whether it involves a paper strip dipped in a cup or a fancy plastic stick you pee on. You'll later blame hCG for your morning sickness, as it similarly peaks around week ten, but for now, its presence in your urine is the most easily detectable early indicator that you are indeed pregnant.

With the proliferation of early detection tests claiming the ability to reveal pregnancy as soon as a week before you miss your period, it's tempting to pull one out the second it is possible to get a positive. However, because hCG levels in urine are low early on, you may get a false negative depending on what time of day you take it and the cycle day. The embryo makes hCG around six to seven days after fertilization during its journey through the fallopian tube toward the uterus. When it implants, hCG production increases quickly, and that is when you are most likely to get an accurate result with at-home tests.

It's highly unlikely you'll receive a false positive unless you are going through fertility treatments, as hCG is rarely produced in detectable levels in the body for any reason other than pregnancy. So even if color on the strip is on the faint side, you are likely pregnant. The main causes of the rare false positive are either not following directions or reading a test incorrectly.

Putting false negatives aside, there is another reason to wait to test. Chemical pregnancies, or very early miscarriages that happen before five weeks, are thought to occur in 50 to 60 percent of all first-time pregnancies and show the same hCG surge. While they can be caused by low hormone levels, inadequate uterine lining, or an infection, most commonly they are tied to chromosomal issues in the embryo. Since the symptoms of a chemical pregnancy are so much like PMS, most women never even know they were pregnant.

How to take a pregnancy test:

- Though it's *really, really* hard, try to wait until your period is due to avoid false negatives and disappointment. If your period is inconsistent, take your first test at least nineteen days after you tried to conceive or believe you ovulated.

- Always take a pregnancy test first thing in the morning, since hCG levels are at their most concentrated before your urine is diluted with coffee or other fluids. For the same reason, don't drink ten glasses of water and then test. If you're testing after five weeks, hCG levels should be high enough to get an accurate result any time of day.

- Read (and follow) the directions on the test you buy. They can be (and often are) confusing. Even though it all seems intuitive (how hard can it be to hold a stick in a stream of urine?), there are actually ways to do it wrong.

- Check the expiration date (the tests become less effective over time).

If you want to confirm the test results or believe a negative result could be wrong, make an appointment with your practitioner or contact a lab and request a beta-hCG test. Beta-hCG tests measure the amount of hCG in the blood, and are more sensitive than urine tests, both because they can detect lower levels and there is more hCG in your blood than your urine. If you're doing IVF, you will go in for a beta-hCG test after your embryo transfer and, pending the results, repeat it a few days later for confirmation the rates are doubling.

IF THINGS GET BUMPY

Understanding fertility issues—
and what to do if you're having one

Sometimes a pregnancy test brings good news, then your period surprises you days or weeks later. Sometimes the opposite is true, and you cannot get pregnant. It's not just a phenomenon for first-time parents: Secondary infertility affects those who have already given birth. If one of these scenarios is true for you, you are in the company of millions who have been there.

If you're nervous reading this section thinking about what could possibly go wrong, take a deep breath. Talking openly about infertility is the best way to remove the shame and secrecy surrounding it. Because even if it doesn't happen to you, someone in your life has gone or is going through it—even if you don't know it yet.

MISCARRIAGE

Miscarriage, or a pregnancy loss before twenty weeks, is known by many names: *early pregnancy loss, fetal demise,* and *spontaneous abortion* among them. After twenty weeks, it's called stillbirth. No matter when it happens, miscarriage can be devastating. While it's hard to remember this if it happens, miscarriage is rarely your fault and is common not only in humans but in other mammal species too.

Many miscarriages happen before a woman knows she's pregnant, and not all are reported, so it's nearly impossible right now to quantify what percentage of total pregnancies end in miscarriage. Our best guess is that it happens in 10 to 20 percent, but the miscarriage rate could be as high as one in three. More than a million women report a miscarriage each year, and 80 percent of these happen in the first trimester. The majority are caused by chromosomal abnormalities, as our body's ability to perform cell division becomes less efficient as we age. This is why the risk of chromosomal issues and miscarriage rises after women hit thirty-five. Men experience fertility decline over forty, too, though chromosomal abnormalities in sperm are a less common cause of miscarriage.

Since it still lives in the shadows, we'll cover a few of the most common miscarriage myths, followed by the top questions people ask when it happens.

Is miscarriage my fault?

Miscarriages can happen no matter how healthy and diligent you are, and though it's very hard not to feel this way, miscarriage is rarely "your fault." The majority are caused by chromosomal abnormalities—not by something you ate or drank, stress, or by working out too hard.

Outside of chromosomal problems, miscarriages can be related to genetic factors, uncontrolled health conditions like diabetes, hormonal and thyroid issues, infections, or uterine or cervical abnormalities. The lifestyle-related factors that you can control are being overweight or underweight, smoking, using drugs, and aggressively consuming alcohol. If you're wondering how to define "aggressive alcohol consumption," miscarriage risk increases 6 percent for each drink you have over five per week.

Why do chromosomal abnormalities happen?

Errors during meiosis, the process that creates eggs and sperm, are the most common cause. Meiotic errors in eggs are responsible for most chromosomal abnormalities that cause miscarriage, birth defects, genetically abnormal pregnancies, and other issues like implantation failure.

An immature egg starts out with two copies of every chromosome and must drop the extras during meiosis before it can be fertilized. During that process, the chromosomes can become misarranged, leaving too few or too many chromosomes in the mature egg. One or more extra or missing chromosomes is called aneuploidy. Aneuploidy is random and unpredictable but happens more frequently with advancing age. Women in their early thirties have an average of 10–25 percent aneuploid eggs; over forty, that number jumps to 50–80 percent.

If I have one miscarriage, will I keep having them?

Fewer than 5 percent of women have two consecutive miscarriages, and only 1 percent experience three or more. Recurrent pregnancy loss is poorly understood but, as the stats indicate, is relatively rare.

If you are concerned about recurrence or just want to talk about why your miscarriage might have happened, make an appointment with your ob-gyn or midwife. It's also a good time to consider making lifestyle adjustments that can improve your overall health. But remember, most miscarriages happen due to chromosomal abnormalities, not something you did wrong, and there was likely nothing you could have done to prevent it.

How can I tell if I'm having a miscarriage?

Spotting and light bleeding around implantation is very common during early pregnancy—one in four women experience it—making it hard to know the difference between that and a miscarriage. If you experience bleeding and any of the below symptoms, it's time to call your physician:

 · Severe abdominal pain
 · Cramps
 · Progression of vaginal bleeding from light to heavy

- Discharge of tissue with clots
- Fever
- Back pain
- Unexplained weakness

There is also a miscarriage type that passes without symptoms: a missed, or silent, miscarriage. Because pregnancy hormones remain the same and a physical miscarriage often doesn't happen for days or even weeks after the embryo or fetus has died, the way most people find out is during an ultrasound when a heartbeat cannot be found.

What do I do if I'm having a miscarriage?

Call your provider. They will ask for the start date of your last period to understand how far along you are, symptoms, and any history of fertility issues. Depending on your circumstances, they may suggest waiting to see if it resolves, ask you to come into the office, or direct you to the emergency room to get checked out. If you cannot reach your provider or someone on call after-hours and the bleeding is heavy, head directly to the ER.

If you do go in, a doctor or nurse will perform an ultrasound to check for an embryo and fetal heartbeat.

How does a miscarriage resolve?

There are several ways. The first is known as *expectant management*, which means letting a miscarriage take a natural course. When a miscarriage happens before nine weeks, most providers take this wait-and-see approach. Given the ever-changing legislative landscape in reproductive health, you may want to understand the options open to you in your state in case of a miscarriage. A first-trimester miscarriage usually feels and looks like a heavy period. Bleeding or passage of tissue should stop in a few hours, and light bleeding typically concludes after several days.

If the miscarriage doesn't or can't clear on its own and it occurs before nine weeks, your doctor will typically prescribe a combination of two medications, mifepristone and misoprostol. They work over a twenty-four-hour period and cause bleeding and intense cramping, and in some cases nausea, vomiting, fever, chills, diarrhea, and headaches. You may not need bed rest but be prepared to take it easy for a few days, and have high-absorbency pads on hand, especially overnight.

If you are nine weeks or more into your pregnancy, a dilation and curettage (D&C) may be performed to remove any remaining tissue. It can be done in an office, in an emergency room, or as a minor outpatient procedure. A D&C takes under thirty minutes and does not require a long recovery period. Your doctor may start the process of dilating your cervix a few hours or the day before the procedure with medication. After it's dilated, the remaining tissue will be removed from your uterus with a long instrument called a curette. You'll spend an hour or two in recovery, so the effects of anesthesia wear off before you leave, and to ensure there is no bleeding. If your blood type is Rh-negative, a shot of RhoGAM will be given, too.

Complications from a D&C are rare, but expect to feel drowsy and have mild cramping and light bleeding afterward. Sex is off-limits for one to two weeks to reduce your infection odds. Your uterus must build a brand-new lining after a D&C, so your period can take longer than one cycle to come back.

When can I try to get pregnant again after a miscarriage?

If the miscarriage happened early and did not require medical intervention to resolve, there is no evidence that shows that waiting even one cycle contributes to the health of future pregnancies. Ovulation can happen as soon as two weeks after a miscarriage, which means you can get pregnant before your period arrives. Most health professionals will tell you that letting yourself heal physically is only half the process, and you should not feel pressured to get pregnant again until you feel ready.

Exactly how many cycles you should wait is best determined by talking to your provider, as it depends on how far along you were when the miscarriage happened, how it resolved, and your overall health.

Opinions range from as soon as you are medically cleared to have sex again to six months, and depend on whether you had a procedure like a D&C and how you recovered.

File under "things we wish we'd known sooner": Fertility doesn't disappear after a miscarriage. Two weeks after mine, the nausea and fatigue returned and, inexplicably, I discovered I was pregnant again. We weren't trying, but we weren't careful, either.

How can I heal emotionally after a miscarriage?

Everyone's reaction to miscarriage is different. Some women are raring to go immediately, and others need time to deal with what happened. Because it wasn't as physically real to them, your partner might process it very differently. Try not to judge if they don't seem to feel it as intensely. Friends and family may not always know what to say or do, so tell them what you need. Same goes for your partner. The answer can be funny cat videos, a night of distraction, or absolutely nothing but the physical presence of another human being. You may be surprised at how many people in your life have had a miscarriage, and that they will mourn the loss with you.

Seeing a therapist or counselor who specializes in processing grief or trauma can also be helpful. Joining a support group allows you to connect with others who have gone through the same loss. Whether you do it in person or online, hearing and reading other people's experiences can be healing, but it can also be triggering, so manage your consumption if it's causing more heartache than help.

I assumed that after decades on the pill our first attempt would be a practice round. Then a few days before my period was due, I woke up feeling like I had the flu. Thinking it couldn't possibly be positive, I took an early detection pregnancy test.
And there they were: two pink lines.

Since we expected conception to take longer, we had scheduled a trip to go skiing in a remote part of British Columbia. Strenuous physical activity was no longer enticing considering my dearth of energy, but I still wanted to go and enjoy the scenery. So the tiny town of Nelson, BC, is where I miscarried.

Far from home, I used Maven, a virtual care platform, to speak with a nurse practitioner, as I had no clue what to do. She advised a trip to the hospital to see if everything was okay. My first trip to the Canadian ER involved an ultrasound and cervix check followed by the first of two blood draws to see if my hCG levels were going up or down. Down meant miscarriage, up meant still pregnant. Based on the volume of bleeding, I knew it was likely bad news, but the twenty-four-hour wait to confirm was still excruciating.

My hCG levels crashed at the follow-up appointment. It was a miscarriage.

Luckily, my body resolved it without any medical intervention. Emotionally, it was less great. I knew logically that the miscarriage wasn't my fault. But there is nothing logical about loss; I felt broken. After I shared what happened with a few friends, several confided that they'd had one, or even more than one. Miscarriage truly is a secret club that no one wants to join, with a member list miles long.

ECTOPIC PREGNANCY

Despite its name, an ectopic pregnancy is not a viable pregnancy. It happens when a fertilized egg grows outside of the uterus, usually in the fallopian tubes. It cannot be moved into the uterus and cannot grow into a healthy fetus. Ectopic pregnancy is dangerous and when detected must be treated immediately, as it can cause the fallopian tubes to rupture, leading to major internal bleeding. If an ectopic is caught before the fallopian tube bursts, it can sometimes be treated with a medication called methotrexate, or it may necessitate surgery. A burst tube requires immediate emergency surgery, as it can be life-threatening.

Risk factors for an ectopic pregnancy are a history of fallopian tube surgery or infertility, pelvic or abdominal surgery, some STIs, pelvic inflammatory disease, endometriosis, smoking, and being over thirty-five. Though ectopics can have some typical pregnancy symptoms, there may be low back and abdominal or pelvic pain, mild cramping on one side, and abnormal vaginal bleeding. Signs that a tube ruptured and it's time to go to the ER are sudden and intense pain in the abdomen or pelvis, weakness, dizziness, fainting, and shoulder pain.

DEALING WITH INFERTILITY

Though, like miscarriage, it still lives largely in the shadows, infertility affects one in six people globally and can manifest as an inability to get or stay pregnant. While women are nearly always treated first, roughly half of all fertility issues are due to problems in men's bodies.

Men's most common fertility problem is related to sperm, especially low count or poor quality. Lifestyle factors like stress, obesity, and smoking reduce sperm count, as do cycling and heat exposure. Male infertility can also be caused by past medical issues or physical impairments like varicocele. But scientists believe the growing number of endocrine-disrupting chemical compounds found in the world around us are also culprits.

Women's fertility issues can be triggered by everything from PCOS to endometriosis, low ovarian reserves, blocked fallopian tubes, a failure to ovulate, and yes, age. While women are born with all the eggs they'll ever have, men make sperm constantly and, with the right adjustments, can often improve their parameters.

If you don't become pregnant right away, remember, it's typically a three-to-six-month process. If you're under thirty-five, a year of unprotected sex that does not end in pregnancy is the guideline before seeking fertility care. If you're over thirty-five, you should talk to your ob-gyn or primary care provider once you hit that six-month mark. If you do, that existing physician will likely refer the two of you to a reproductive endocrinologist, an ob-gyn who specifically treats infertility.

At your first appointment (please go together), they will talk about your medical history and lifestyle and run a few tests. Their questions and recommendations will be related to things like whether you are having regular periods, eating well, are over- or underweight, exercising, smoking, or using recreational drugs, and ensuring none of your medications interfere with your fertility.

When it comes to tests for women, here are the initial candidates:
- Everyone's favorite—the Pap smear
- A blood test during your period to check for hormone imbalances, especially FSH (follicle-stimulating hormone), LH (luteinizing hormone), and estradiol
- A blood test to confirm you are ovulating during your fertile window
- A urine test for chlamydia (its presence can block your fallopian tubes)

If the clinic does not bring up testing for your partner, demand it. Because even if there is an issue on your end, there may be something going on with him, too. When (not if!) your partner gets tested, here are their first steps:
- A urine test for chlamydia, which affects sperm function
- A semen analysis to check for abnormal sperm shapes or poor motility
- Pending the results of the semen analysis, they may also undergo further blood tests, a testicular biopsy, or a karyotype to determine if there are any chromosomal abnormalities.

If the results are inconclusive after your first visit, your doctor will run further diagnostics. These can include:

- A more extensive hormone panel to measure any other possible imbalances
- An ultrasound to look at your uterus and ovaries
- A series of ultrasound scans to see if or how many antral follicles, the small sacs of fluid in the ovary that mature and release eggs, are developing over time
- A hysterosalpingogram, a procedure that uses X-ray imaging to confirm your fallopian tubes are open and working
- A hysteroscopy, a procedure that allows your doctor to look inside your uterus with a camera to check for fibroids and polyps
- Genetic testing, as there are screens for fertility-related risk factors that allow a more personalized treatment plan.

Sometimes there are no answers, and between 15 and 30 percent of couples are diagnosed with unexplained infertility. This lack of diagnosis can lead people to obsess over or doubt test results or to believe something more serious is wrong. Suboptimal test results are also possible, and frustrating because they don't preclude spontaneous pregnancy but also do not explain why you aren't getting pregnant.

FERTILITY TREATMENTS

The goal of fertility treatment is to start with less invasive, less expensive options before moving on to IVF unless it's indicated. These treatments can include medications like Clomid, which are prescribed for ovulatory issues or to stimulate testosterone or sperm production. Timed intercourse can pinpoint your exact ovulatory window and involves ultrasound monitoring of your follicular development and then sex every day or every other day during a precisely timed window.

We talked about intracervical (ICI) or intravaginal insemination (IVI) earlier. Both can be done at home with an FDA-cleared kit and are designed to deposit sperm into the vagina near the cervix, which is then held in place with a cervical cap or menstrual cup. This allows sperm concentration in the cervical mucus to be higher than traditional intercourse since it doesn't have to navigate the vagina's obstacle course. Unlike intrauterine insemination (IUI), these methods are much cheaper, as they simulate what happens during sex, and insertion stops at the cervix instead of going all the way into the uterus. The efficacy is similar to IUI, and it is a fraction of the cost. IVI is also useful if you're struggling to conceive but haven't hit the six- or twelve-month timeline to go to a clinic or, yes, are sick of timed sex.

IUI

Most treatments in a clinic and anyone conceiving with donor sperm start with intrauterine insemination (IUI). IUI closes the time and distance sperm have to travel to the egg by depositing sperm directly into the uterus during ovulation. It also uses a sperm sample that has been filtered for the strongest swimmers. It is done if you have unexplained infertility, diminished ovarian reserves, PCOS, or an irregular cycle, or if sperm are of low motility or quality. Some women need fertility medications to help things along or hormones to trigger ovulation, too.

A sperm sample goes through a process called *washing* to ensure that only the healthy, motile specimens remain. The sample is then inserted through the cervix and directly into the uterus around the time of ovulation via a thin tube. Insemination takes only five to ten minutes at your doctor's office, or in a fertility clinic, and doesn't require any anesthesia. Some people report cramping, but otherwise the whole process is pretty painless. If the sperm and egg come together, and the fertilized embryo implants in your uterus, you're pregnant.

IUI is the most affordable place to start exploring alternative conception methods, at $500 to $4,000 per session. Success rates are between 5 and 20 percent per cycle, and it's most likely to work during the first three or four treatments.

IVF

On July 25, 1978, Louise Brown came into the world at Royal Oldham Hospital in the UK. As the first baby conceived and born via in vitro fertilization (IVF), she paved the way for the more than twelve million IVF babies born around the world since.

IVF is used in women with blocked or damaged fallopian tubes, ovulation disorders, or uterine fibroids; when a woman's partner has decreased sperm count or motility; when one or both partners have a genetic disorder; or if there is unexplained infertility. It can be done with your egg and your partner's sperm, or with donor sperm and eggs, and can involve a gestational carrier or surrogate.

Women who have been through IVF often describe it as an emotional and hormonal roller coaster, due to the high costs and uncertainty, not to mention the effects of the daily shots that actually pump you full of hormones. It's also not without risks. IVF increases the likelihood of multiple births, miscarriage odds climb to 15 to 25 percent, and 2 to 5 percent of women have an ectopic pregnancy.

IVF starts with an examination of the ovaries and hormone level checks, and, pending results, fertility medications to stimulate egg production are prescribed. After a few weeks, eggs are retrieved through a minor surgical procedure that uses ultrasound imaging to guide a hollow needle through the pelvic cavity. You may feel a little sore or bruised and have cramps and spotting after the retrieval. At the same time, your partner contributes a sperm sample which will be analyzed and prepared.

The work is handled by embryologists, or the lab scientists who create embryos for implantation. They start by isolating the sperm from the semen, and the eggs from the ovarian fluid. Then, the egg and sperm are combined, and the resulting fertilized eggs are sent to an incubator to develop. Each embryo is monitored and checked during development and tested for chromosomal abnormalities when indicated or requested. If an embryo makes the grade, it is transferred or frozen to be used later.

Your fertility clinic will tailor treatments specifically to your needs, but with few exceptions, specialists recommend single embryo transfer to avoid risks associated with multiple births. The transfer itself starts just like a Pap smear, as the physician will use a speculum to gain access to the cervix. A fine tube is passed through the cervix using ultrasound guidance, and the embryos are inserted into the uterus. Outside of Pap smear–level discomfort, it's relatively painless.

If the cycle is successful, implantation occurs six to ten days after an egg retrieval during the dreaded two-week wait.

Your physician or friends may have fertility clinic recommendations, but if you'd like to do your own research, the Society for Assisted Reproductive Technology (SART) includes data on over 90 percent of reproductive clinics, or you can consult the CDC's yearly Assisted Reproductive Technology (ART) report. While this data can be helpful, it isn't perfect. A clinic's success rates can vary year to year based on how many cycles were performed. More cycles equal more consistent stats over time. Also, some clinics refuse treatment for poor-prognosis patients to boost their stats, and clinics that appear to have lower rates of positive outcomes are often willing to take on more complex cases.

DONORS AND SURROGACY

Gamete donation

When one or both partners cannot provide their own egg or sperm, usually due to poor quality or the risk of passing down genetic disorders, gamete donation makes it possible to experience pregnancy and birth and, when possible, allows one partner to maintain a genetic connection to the baby.

Donor material can be sourced from reproductive centers, donor agencies and banks, or from family members and friends. Before a donor is accepted, they go through a health screening that includes medical history, genetic risks, STDs, and a physical. There are long-term ramifications of genetic connections, so the screening also includes a psychological component, and counseling for both the donor and intended parents is highly recommended. The donor's motivations can vary, especially if it is someone who will be part of the child's life, so it's best to understand them before moving forward. As intended parents, you should think about how you will eventually tell your child that they do not share your genetic makeup, as, with today's ancestry and consumer genetics testing, keeping this fact a secret is impossible. Most parents now choose to make it a part of their child's story from the very beginning.

Legally, an agreement will be put in place outlining everyone's roles, obligations, and expectations. This includes everything from financial arrangements to possible future contact and is especially important if the donor is someone you know. Parentage laws for the donor and intended parents vary by state and even county, so clarify and paper everything with legal counsel if you start down this path.

Surrogacy and gestational carriers

The number of births that involve a gestational carrier or surrogate has more than doubled since 2013. The reasons are myriad that a woman cannot carry a baby to term—life-threatening congenital abnormalities, a nonfunctional or missing uterus (yes, some women are born without one), conditions like pulmonary hypertension, cancer treatments, or more than five pregnancy losses. Surrogacy and gestational carriers are also options for LGBTQ couples or single parents.

You may be wondering why anyone would sign up for the job of carrying someone else's child. The reasons can be financially moti-vated but are also usually personal, and if you interview a few, you'll find everyone has a different answer. What they share is a love of either all or some part of the pregnancy experience, combined with a desire to help prospective parents achieve their dream of building a family. Many cite family members or friends who experienced fertility issues and, having had an easy delivery themselves, a wish to pay it forward.

How do you decide which is right for you? If you have embryos ready to transfer via IVF, a gestational carrier is your best bet. If your eggs cannot be used, choosing between a surrogate or gestational car-rier comes down to deciding where the egg comes from.

A gestational carrier becomes pregnant via IVF and has a gesta-tional relationship but no genetic relationship with the embryo. A sur-rogate traditionally uses her own eggs, fertilized via IUI or IVF with your partner's or a donor's sperm, meaning she has a genetic and ges-tational relationship.

Candidates should be between the ages of twenty-one and forty, have had at least one uncomplicated pregnancy, no more than three cesarean deliveries and no more than five pregnancies total, and no chronic medical conditions. A psychological screening is also impor-tant, especially with surrogates, as there is a genetic link. This means addressing any religious and ethical views that could complicate the handoff of the infant later.

Cost is a big consideration, as no matter where you do it the total is $100,000 or more. You can find one through agencies, IVF clinics, specialized attorneys, and online. This raises another essential aspect: putting a legally binding contract into place. You and the surrogate or carrier must have your own separate legal representation, then agree to terms regarding the pregnancy and your designation as the legal parents. If the cost or complication of finding someone puts this option out of reach, family members sometimes volunteer. Consider this carefully before agreeing, as it can be much more emotionally complex than enlisting a stranger.

Trimester-Zero Checklist

☐   Start taking prenatal vitamins at least three months before you try to conceive (both of you!).

☐   Clean up your lifestyles.

☐   Schedule preconception checkups.

☐   Get necessary immunizations if you're not up-to-date.

☐   Check the safety of your prescription medications and compatibility with fertility and pregnancy.

☐   Quit birth control and get to know your cycle.

☐   Talk about your parenting goals.

☐   Try not to make having sex a job.

☐   Sleep, eat moderately, and move your body.

The First Trimester

Now that you're pregnant—or reading ahead—let's get a few things out of the way.

You probably won't look like a celebrity traipsing breezily across the pages of *Vogue* in a flawless maternity ensemble. You will not wake up every day feeling or looking great. You might experience the joys of morning sickness, back pain, fatigue, and all the rest. Or you might not.

You may relish every moment of pregnancy and the new and interesting changes to your body. Or, *you may not like being pregnant.* Many women don't!

But even if you follow what your doctor and everyone else recommends to the letter, your pregnancy will not be perfect.

To all you fellow type As out there, if conception didn't already teach you this lesson, now is the time to grow comfortable with the idea that you are not in full control of this process. Pregnancy is great training for parenting because no matter what you do, *things will not always go the way you expect.* More opinions and data are not always better—sometimes they're just more. And the more you obsess over every micro decision, the crazier you will drive yourself.

I put my ulcerative colitis (UC, a type of irritable bowel disorder) into remission with the help of connected devices and a food and lifestyle diary kept over a year. A decade later, my UC is still under control, so long as I avoid my triggers.

So if I could kick UC into remission, why not use similar micromanagement methods during pregnancy to handle the mass of crazy happening to my body?

Rookie move. I tried dozens of apps and services to diligently track my symptoms and weight and get updates on the baby's size and development the first two times I was pregnant. Unlike managing my gut problems, none of it improved my symptoms at all, and frankly, it stoked some unhealthy obsessive tendencies. The content brought up all the things that could go wrong, and what should be happening each day, and when it didn't match exactly, I panicked.

There can be huge differences between pregnancies—even in the same person, even if they are close together and you do exactly the same things.

When I became pregnant for the third time, I continued to make healthy choices, but also chose to chill out and try to just listen to my body and minimized content consumption. Key word chose, *as I woke up every day and mindfully managed my thoughts. Instead of living with a persistent drumbeat of silent worry, I talked about it. Letting go made the whole experience much more enjoyable, and as the pregnancy progressed, my anxiety (mostly) faded.*

This pregnancy was nothing like the first two. No nausea, my fatigue level was a 5 instead of a 9, and I felt more like myself. The first trimester whizzed by. We navigated the gauntlet of tests and appointments as best we could, though it was still difficult not to sometimes imagine all the things that could go wrong.

So, as you head into this brave new world, remember that every pregnancy is different. Every pregnant body is different. Yours will be different if you get pregnant again. And sometimes pregnancy feels like an amazing, magical cruise gliding toward the destination of your dreams. Other times it feels like a hijacking— of your body, your mind, and your freedom.

SO WHAT'S HAPPENING IN THERE?

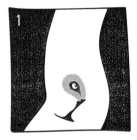 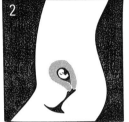 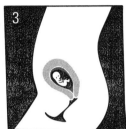

Month 1

Baby: The first month of pregnancy starts with your period, which is an important data point. It may sound strange, but the first day of your last menstrual period (LMP) is when the clock starts on pregnancy, and how your provider will calculate your estimated due date. For the first two weeks, your uterus is playing the waiting game until ovulation and thickening its lining. Once the egg and sperm meet during week three, they'll start the fertilization process, and the resulting cell will begin to divide and implant into the uterine lining in week four. The amniotic and yolk sacs are also forming at the end of the first month, and the brand-new embryo is around the size of a poppy seed.

You: Think of month one as a bonus month. Most symptoms don't start until around six weeks, but as we've established, every pregnancy (and person) is different. You may have spotting around implantation, which is typically six to twelve days after you conceive. Fatigue, more frequent trips to the restroom, breast tenderness, and morning sickness can show up toward the end of this month, though outside of bloating and fuller breasts, you will probably look about the same.

Month 2

Baby: The embryo is growing at a rapid clip—in fact, by the end of the fifth week the cardiac muscle that will later be a heart is the size of a poppy seed. The embryonic period, which spans weeks five to ten, is all about establishing the foundations of the major systems, including the neural tube (the future spinal cord and brain), the circulatory system, the kidneys, the lungs, the mouth, the eyes, and the arm and leg buds. The embryo will close out week eight around the size of that prenatal vitamin you've been taking every day.

You: Month two can be a tough one. Symptoms and surging hormones can wreak havoc on your emotions, which may be all over the place now that the reality of pregnancy is setting in. Morning sickness and other digestion-related issues may start, along with fatigue, headaches, frequent peeing, and breast changes. No symptoms? Consider yourself lucky, as feeling normal is normal, too. You may start to notice your clothes getting tighter, as your uterus has grown from the size of a fist to that of a roll of toilet paper.

Month 3

Baby: The embryo kicks off this month around the size of the tip of your index finger and will officially earn the rank of fetus in week eleven. Hair follicles, nail beds, bones, cartilage, and muscles are forming, allowing arm and leg movement along-side the beginnings of digestion and hormone production. It is also time for your first prenatal appointment, where you'll hear the heartbeat for the first time. It's an incredible moment— enjoy. By the close of week thirteen, a.k.a. the end of the first trimester, the fetus will be about the size of a baseball.

You: If you are experiencing the pains of pregnancy symptoms like morning sickness, this month is when they usually peak. Take solace that when you enter the second trimester, you'll start to feel better. Vacillating between irritable, irrational, and joyful is completely normal, as is bursting into tears over cute baby animals. But if you find your downs far outnumber your ups, depression during pregnancy is a symptom to address early. After week ten, morning sickness and aversions can start to diminish, and your appetite may pick up. Your waist will start to get thicker, meaning the days of wearing your prepregnancy pants without getting creative are numbered.

SYMPTOMS AND SOLUTIONS

While the saying "eating for two" isn't accurate, sleeping for two almost certainly will be. Many women describe the first trimester as the worst trimester for two reasons: You won't look pregnant for a while, so nice side effects like strangers giving up subway seats or lifting your bag into the overhead bin are unlikely. And since you probably aren't telling the whole world yet, you will suffer much of this in silence. Hang on—it gets better.

The severity and prevalence of symptoms are impossible to predict. Some people experience all of them; a lucky few have none. Most are somewhere in the middle. While you're in the throes, just remember: As miserable as they can be, it's all temporary. However, if you have any of these symptoms, call your doctor:

- Vaginal bleeding
- Persistent vomiting
- Blurred vision
- Chills or fever
- Headache that doesn't resolve with water or acetaminophen

- Sudden swelling of hands or face
- Fluid leaking from vagina

My first two pregnancies were nauseous miseries. Like my mom before me, I never actually threw up, but man did I want to. Sniffing lemon and mint helped, but it was still unbearable. My third was blissfully free of morning sickness, but my reflux was constant, from positive test through birth, and worse after.

Super smell was also a struggle, especially while enclosed with odorous people and things. Worst of all were car air fresheners. I had to stick my head out the window like a dog just to make it through one rush-hour ride.

FOR PARTNERS

Though it will be all about Mom for the next nine months (then all about the baby after that), finding out you're expecting is a huge transitional time for you as well. Your partner doesn't have much control over what's happening in there and might sometimes feel like a different person. The raging hormones, physical transformations, and abundance of unsolicited advice she'll receive for the next nine months can be overwhelming. She may not always know how or want to ask for help, which is why you have to take more initiative. Here are a few simple ways to get started.

Ask what she needs

Pregnancy brings on brand-new emotions, stress, and occasional (sometimes frequent!) out-of-character behavior. Don't assume you know how she feels or what she needs. Ask, listen, and be prepared to act on whatever she says. Even if she demands something gross, like a sauerkraut-and-banana sandwich.

Remind her she's beautiful and loved

A pregnant body is a miraculous, beautiful thing. That does not mean that all women feel miraculous or beautiful while pregnant, especially in the later stages. Don't be shy about telling her often how much you love her. Share your excitement and help her overcome self-consciousness related to physical changes.

Become a pregnancy pro

Though you aren't actually pregnant, you can follow along and mentally prepare for how her body will change, the challenges she will face, and when and how her energy will fluctuate. Stepping up especially during the times of greatest change to help around the house or do something kind (foot rubs, date nights, food runs, letting her have the run of the Netflix account) can make a world of difference.

Attend and take notes during doctor's appointments

The idea of a growing baby inside a woman's body is an abstract concept—until you hear a heartbeat during the first ultrasound. Attending doctor's appointments makes everything feel more real, and it's an opportunity for you to pitch in while she's covered in goo or being poked and prodded. Take notes, and make sure you have a record of follow-up or action items. For extra points, keep a note on your phone about questions the two of you have between appointments so nothing slips. Even if your practitioner sends you after-visit notes, you'll be surprised by how much information you immediately forget.

First-trimester symptoms and solutions

Morning sickness (a.k.a. all-day sickness)

- **When does it happen?**
  Typically starts around week 5 or 6, peaks around 9 or 10, then disappears in your second trimester

- **Symptoms**
  Nausea, vomiting, aversions to foods and certain smells, cravings

- **Cause**
  Caused by rising levels of pregnancy hormones, scientists suspect it evolved to prevent dangerous substances and our varied diets from hurting development, as it occurs primarily when the baby's core organ systems are formed.

- **Solutions**
  Eat small meals and snacks slowly and frequently, drink fluids between meals, and avoid trigger smells. Acupuncture, sipping mint- or citrus-flavored water, enjoying ginger tea or chews, using acupressure bands, and taking a walk can also help.

Fatigue

- **When does it happen?**
  One of the earliest symptoms that persists in the first and third trimesters and subsides during the second

- **Symptoms**
  Falling asleep in the middle of the afternoon, craving a 7:00 p.m. bedtime, inability to pry yourself out of bed in the morning

- **Cause**
Sky-high progesterone levels

- **Solutions**
Eat healthy foods (avoid processed and packaged foods), try to get some exercise, take walks and breathe in the fresh air, sleep.

Gas and bloating

- **When does it happen?**
Can start immediately or closer to the start of the second trimester

- **Symptoms**
Gas, bloating, feeling like your abdomen is inflated like a bicycle tire

- **Cause**
Progesterone causes the gastrointestinal tract to relax, slowing down digestion so nutrients can enter the bloodstream and reach your baby.

- **Solutions**
Eat more fiber, take your time and eat smaller meals, up your water-drinking game.

Heartburn and reflux

- **When does it happen?**
Can start immediately or in the second and third trimesters, when things begin getting more crowded

- Symptoms

  Burning sensation in your throat or chest, and/or the taste of bile after a meal

- Cause

  Surging progesterone levels relax the valve between your stomach and esophagus, allowing bile to travel back up.

- Solutions

  Eat smaller, more frequent meals; avoid acidic foods like citrus and tomatoes, fatty, oily, fried and spicy foods, and caffeine; do not lie down right after a meal.

Food aversions and cravings

- When does it happen?

  Can persist throughout pregnancy but lessen in the third trimester

- Symptoms

  Sensitivity to odors and changing taste preferences

- Cause

  Hormonal changes

- Solutions

  Keep serving sizes small when indulging in unhealthy cravings, or distract yourself if ice cream dreams are all-consuming. If vegetables sound or smell terrible, try blending them into a smoothie with fruit to hide the offending texture or taste.

Tender or swollen breasts

- **When does it happen?**
  Can be one of the first pregnancy symptoms; acute symptoms typically diminish in a few weeks but will persist on and off throughout pregnancy.

- **Symptoms**
  Sore or sensitive breasts and nipples

- **Cause**
  Hormonal changes

- **Solutions**
  Avoid the shower spray and other unnecessary contact, get fitted for a new bra, or transition into a sports or nursing bra.

Acne

- **When does it happen?**
  Mostly the first and second trimesters

- **Symptoms**
  Teenage-style breakouts that can happen all over your body

- **Cause**
  Progesterone. Again. Also fluid retention.

- **Solutions**
  Eat well, drink water, and keep your face, body, and hair clean. Do not use spot treatments that contain salicylic acid.

Peeing all the damn time

- **When does it happen?**
  Another early pregnancy symptom that peaks around weeks 6 to 8. Will lessen by the end of the first trimester, then pick up again in the third with the increased pressure on your bladder.

- **Symptoms**
  Needing the loo urgently throughout the day and several (many?) times in the middle of the night

- **Cause**
  Increased blood volume in your body causes kidneys to process extra fluid that goes into your bladder.

- **Solutions**
  Stop drinking liquids a few hours before bedtime. Lean forward when you pee to make sure you're really done. Regulate caffeine intake.

Constipation

- **When does it happen?**
  Can be one of the first pregnancy symptoms, will persist throughout pregnancy

- **Symptoms**
  Cramping, bloating, farting, gassiness, and inability to poop

- **Cause**
  Those pesky high-progesterone levels slowing down your digestive system

- Solutions

Drink plenty of fluids, up your fiber intake, and exercise. Avoid laxatives, which can cause dehydration or uterine contractions. MiraLAX or a generic equivalent is the safe exception. Find ways to relax—stress makes it worse!

Super smell

- When does it happen?

Early pregnancy symptom that can persist until birth

- Symptoms

Ability to smell anything from across a room more vividly. Unearthly aversion to cigarette smell.

- Cause

Estrogen

- Solutions

Carry products scented with citrus (especially lemon) or mint and sniff as needed. Put baking soda in your refrigerator. Make your partner take out the trash. Stay out of enclosed spaces.

PREGNANCY FAQ, LIGHTNING ROUND

Bite-size answers to everything you secretly wonder about pregnancy (but are too afraid to ask)

Inevitably, you've started trolling the internet for answers to pregnancy questions large and small. When you spend enough time in forums (and it really doesn't take long!), you'll run into some kooks. If it hasn't happened yet, get ready to be pummeled with anecdotes, uninformed (yet strong) opinions, and bad science.

To protect your sanity, below are the most popular pregnancy questions answered with scientific evidence. They range from things you might be too embarrassed to ask, like does sleeping on your stomach crush the baby (nope!) and can I still have sex (yep!), to topics like how to prevent stretch marks (you can't!) and what are those brown splotches on my cheeks (ack, melasma!)?

OMG I accidentally had too many cocktails right before I found out I was pregnant! Did I hurt my baby?

You're not alone, especially if you're taking a laissez-faire approach to getting pregnant, or it was unplanned. If your main concern is fetal alcohol syndrome, it is typically associated with heavy drinking during an entire pregnancy, not a one-time event.

A rager before your missed period is unlikely to cause any lasting or major harm. If it had, it probably would have ended as a miscarriage before you ever knew you were pregnant. If it happened in the first weeks after a missed period, there is more risk, though it's still small. If you are concerned, talk to your doctor.

What do you mean my doctor won't see me until I'm eight to ten weeks pregnant?!

Yes, it's true—most care providers require that you be at least eight weeks in before your first appointment. Sometimes it's ten. It's hard to see much on the ultrasound before that time or do anything other than confirm the pregnancy with a blood test.

If you have a complicated medical history, are on medications with possible side effects, are otherwise high risk (e.g., diabetes, high blood pressure, seizure disorder), or just really can't wait that long, some providers will make an exception and see you earlier.

Do I have to stop baths, steam rooms, hot tubs, saunas, and (gasp) hot yoga while I'm pregnant?

When your core body temperature is too elevated, it causes a condition called hyperthermia, which can be dangerous during pregnancy. The main issue: There are several (admittedly limited) studies that show a connection between neural tube defects and time in hot tubs during the first trimester. Spending time in an enclosed heated space or immersed in hot water also makes pregnancy symptoms like dizziness and light-headedness worse, which can lead to falls and other injuries.

If you want the more detailed version, here you go: Since hot tubs are typically set to 104 degrees Fahrenheit, and saunas are even hotter, it takes only ten to twenty minutes for your body to heat up to 102 degrees Fahrenheit, which is the magic core temperature pregnancy research suggests avoiding. Your warm nightly bath or morning shower is fine, since your entire body isn't covered, but the water temperature shouldn't take an adjustment period; it should be comfortable immediately.

To be safe, avoid anything that would cause you to overheat in the first trimester, and if you indulge in a steam or sauna in the second or third, keep your visits short.

How do I figure out my due date?

It's really best to look at it as a due-date *range*, since only about 5 percent of babies arrive on the day they are expected. That said, there are a few ways to calculate your estimated due date (EDD). The most common: Add seven days to the first day of your last period, then count nine months forward. Or take the route of less math: Your EDD is forty weeks after the first day of your last period. There are loads of due date calculators online that will do the heavy lifting for you if you supply your LMP.

An ultrasound at eleven to fourteen weeks is another way your practitioner may date the pregnancy, although it's less common. This method can be more precise if ovulation happened on a different cycle day. But don't expect the EDD to change as your pregnancy continues. Even though they will take some measurements during ultrasounds, your practitioner will likely stick with the first-trimester date, as it's more accurate.

Can I have sex while I'm pregnant?

Sure can! Sex will not hurt the baby, and the baby will not see anything requiring therapy later. The better question is what your sex drive will be like. Often it dips in the blah first trimester, comes back raging in the second (increased blood flow down there! More energy!), then goes back down in the third, when the bump gets in the way of pretty much everything. It's best to just pay attention, relax, and go with what feels good at the time.

The exception: If you have a high-risk pregnancy (e.g., placenta previa or shortened cervix) and your provider cautions against it or puts you on pelvic rest. Same if you have pain during sex.

What if I don't have any symptoms, or they stop?

Feel fortunate and enjoy it! If symptoms stop and aren't accompanied by anything else like bleeding or cramping, it doesn't mean you aren't pregnant anymore, or that something is wrong. Morning sickness, discomfort, hormonal surges, and the like come and go. Their absence or presence doesn't predict an empty ultrasound at your next prenatal appointment.

I am puking so much that I can't leave the house; I'm dizzy and losing weight. Is this normal?

Eighty percent of pregnant women with morning sickness say they experience nausea or vomiting all day. Both are common pregnancy symptoms, usually starting at six or eight weeks and mostly disappearing after twelve weeks.

A more serious form of this experience, hyperemesis gravidarum, affects 3 percent of pregnant women and can last a whole pregnancy. The most common symptoms of hyperemesis are vomiting three or more times per day, losing 5 percent or more of your prepregnancy weight, dehydration, dizziness, peeing less than normal, headaches, and fainting. It is caused by a hormone called GDF15, and women with little exposure to it prepregnancy are most likely to experience severe symptoms. Call your provider if the above symptoms are severe or if you cannot stay hydrated. There are medications that can help, or you can also try lifestyle changes like eating small meals consisting of bland foods and avoiding triggers like car rides whenever possible.

When can I tell people I'm pregnant?

No right answer to this one. Most people wait to tell anyone but close friends and family until after the twelve-week mark, when the risk of miscarriage drops. Others who've had more complicated journeys may wait until after the twenty-week anatomy scan, when they feel assured everything is okay to share widely. Still others can't wait to break the news to the whole world and post their positive pregnancy tests. If this is you, just be sure that you are equipped to field questions if anything goes wrong.

When it comes to work, again, it's personal. Most people choose to wait to tell a boss or coworkers until the second trimester. If your work involves heavy-duty physical activity that you can no longer do, you need to share sooner. Same if you have any complications.

I have to commute and spend all day in an office and it is so hard to act normal with all of these pregnancy symptoms. Any hacks for how to cope?

This dynamic is another reason that the first trimester really is the worst trimester. You're not showing, no one knows, and you feel terrible. If you can make a call a walking call or a meeting a stroll, fresh air helps. If you're too tired, try to keep your schedule as light as you can and take breaks throughout the day. Pack snacks and keep things you like at your desk. If things are really bad, open up to a coworker you trust or, if you need to, your boss.

When will I feel the baby moving?

You have a little while before this happens. Most first-time mothers feel movement—also called the quickening—around eighteen to twenty weeks. If this is not your first pregnancy, it can be as soon as thirteen to sixteen weeks. The timing can vary widely, so don't worry if it's not on that exact timeline.

You also may not even realize it's happening, as the first twinges are subtle. They feel like flutters, or even just gas or indigestion. In time you will recognize kicks and punches and be able to detect a distinct pattern and schedule as you move into the third trimester. And toward the end, you'll wish for a break from the rib kicks and middle-of-the-night hiccups.

> *Yes, feeling your baby move is amazing and surreal. Growing a human being inside your body is also really weird to contemplate. My third trimester was spent dealing with contraction-causing kicks to the ribs and hiccups every night at 3:00 a.m. Both were aggressive enough to wake me up, and only pacing and jiggling around made them stop.*

Why is my skin changing color?

The culprit: skin cells called melanocytes. Their job is to produce melanin, the pigment that causes you to tan in the sun. The surges of estrogen and progesterone during pregnancy cause melanocytes to kick into overdrive and produce more melanin where they are most concentrated, like areas with previous skin damage, your areolas, and the connective tissue that goes down the middle of your stomach. During pregnancy, this brown line bisecting your belly, also known as the linea nigra, becomes more prominent, especially with sun exposure. It fades in the months after birth.

The other common skin issue is melasma, or "the mask of pregnancy." It appears as dark patches on your face, especially the forehead, nose, and cheeks. These skin issues will mostly resolve a few months after birth or when you conclude breastfeeding, so skip the lightening creams and laser treatments until your pregnant years are over.

Is pregnancy brain real?

Sorry, can you repeat the question?

As pregnancy wears on, you may notice your ability to communicate or remember what you had for breakfast diminishes. Fun fact: Your brain shrinks during pregnancy and doesn't return to its original size until two years postpartum. We don't really know why. But the loss of gray matter doesn't mean you are getting dumber. The theory is that the contraction makes the brain more efficient in responding to your baby's needs and increases maternal attachment.

What's with all the peeing?

The culprit: the hormone hCG, as it increases the blood flow to your kidneys and pelvic area. Frequent peeing starts around the time you miss your period; gets better during the second trimester, when the uterus rises and takes pressure off your bladder; and is even more frequent in the final weeks of the third trimester, when the baby's head drops back on your bladder. Don't avoid water or fluids, as pregnancy puts women at increased risk of UTIs and it's much easier to get dehydrated.

How do I prevent stretch marks?

Skip the expensive lotions, creams, and brews promising a perfectly smooth postpartum belly. Getting stretch marks (or not) is largely a function of genetics. If your mom had them during pregnancy, or if you already have a history of stretch marks, you may also get them. Stretch marks also happen when your skin can't keep up with how quickly your body is expanding. So outside of being born with the right genes, gaining weight gradually is your best defense.

No amount of cocoa butter or fancy oils can prevent stretch marks entirely, but they can help make them less obvious and relieve the itching from your growing bump. Bonus: Slathering on lotion is a nice way to feel pampered and rubbing it on your legs and ankles can help promote better circulation.

I don't want to wait to learn the gender! How can I find out now?

Read enough forums and you'll find plenty of ways to "predict" gender early. These include the Ramzi method (based on chromosome polarity—if early ultrasounds show the placenta forming on the right side of your body, it's a boy, left it's a girl), how you're carrying (belly it's a boy, hips it's a girl), length of linea nigra (if it stops at your belly button, it's a girl, all the way to your ribs it's a boy), fetal heart rate (over 140 means a girl, under means a boy), and Chinese and Mayan birth tables. Though it can be tempting to try them all, there is no proof that any are accurate.

The earliest way to definitively learn gender is the noninvasive prenatal screening (NIPS) at ten weeks in your doctor's office. It looks for common chromosomal conditions through the fetal DNA circulating in your blood and also detects male and female chromosomes. There are kits available online that promise to do the same thing as early as six weeks, but the longer you wait, the more likely you are to get the correct answer.

If you are pursuing diagnostic testing, chorionic villus sampling (CVS) can also provide answers at ten to thirteen weeks, amniocentesis at fifteen to twenty weeks, or if you wait until your anatomy ultrasound at eighteen to twenty-two weeks, the genitalia (helllloooo penis!) is developed enough to be visible. There are risks with CVS and amnio, so if those tests aren't indicated and you aren't eligible for or opt out of NIPS (it's ordered automatically if you're over thirty-five), be patient and wait until the anatomy scan.

Will sleeping on my stomach squash the baby?

No. Stomach sleeping will become very uncomfortable as your pregnancy wears on, but the amniotic sac provides plenty of cushion so your baby doesn't turn into a pancake.

Trust me—you won't even want to sleep on your stomach. What you will want is one of those extremely unsexy wraparound body pillows so you and your bump can get some rest. I wanted to torch mine by the end (my water broke all over it, so instead of ritual burning it just went in the trash), but it was a lifesaver in getting sleep from the middle of the second trimester to birth.

Will lying on my back hurt the baby?

There is no evidence that you will harm the baby or cause a stillbirth by sleeping on your back. However, it may make you dizzy and want to turn over. The added weight of the baby and their home and accessories compresses the vein that carries blood from the lower half of your body up the right side to your heart. For this reason, many women prefer their left side starting at around twenty weeks, as lying on the right sometimes has a similar effect.

Will my nose spread and feet grow an extra size?

Feet can grow during pregnancy and stay that way, thanks to the extra weight you cart around for almost a year, and to the effects of the hormone relaxin. And yes, your nose can too, courtesy of the increased estrogen-related blood flow to your mucous membranes, with more rhinitis and postnasal drip. Luckily, that one is temporary and your nose will revert back to its original size after you give birth. But there is one other surprise change later: an expanded rib cage, also caused by relaxin. This one can take years to train back.

Why shouldn't I change my cat's litter box?

While it's more connected with eating uncooked and cured meats, the issue is an infection called toxoplasmosis, which can be passed through your purring ball of love's feces to your growing baby. It's uncommon in full-grown indoor cats, but if you are around three or more kittens while you are pregnant, your odds of infection increase. It's unlikely to be an issue—in fact, you're more likely to contract it by eating raw and undercooked meats—but hey, pregnancy is a great excuse to hand off poop-scooping responsibilities.

Wait, I shouldn't garden either?

Working with soil is a more likely source of toxoplasmosis than emptying the kitty litter and one reason why also involves feline friends. If your flower beds are a haven for the bathroom activities of neighborhood cats, the parasites excreted by those infected with toxoplasmosis can live for up to a year in the water or dirt. So if your nesting instinct inspired you to plant a vegetable garden, wear gloves, and wash everything that comes out of it thoroughly. Same goes for produce in general—if it grows in the ground, give it an extra rinse before you eat it.

Should I keep my laptop away from my bump? What about my cell phone?

Don't pull out the tinfoil hat yet. We don't really know how or even if cellular signals or wireless connections affect your unborn child, as (drumroll, please) subjecting a fetus or pregnant woman to the risks of that research is ethically questionable.

The electromagnetic waves our devices send and receive are absorbed into our bodies in tiny amounts and, as far as we know, don't cause any harm. In high doses (like, *really* high doses), they can cause damage. Airplanes, the sun, and your microwave also emit electromagnetic waves, so unless you are going to live in a cave for nine months, there is no way to avoid all of it completely.

If you can't help but worry, keep your cell phone away from your midsection, and do not put it near you next to the bed while you sleep. Put it in airplane mode for extra points. Laptop enthusiasts, try not to use your bump as a desk, especially if your computer heats up.

What if I get sick while I'm pregnant?

Managing a virus or any illness while pregnant is no fun. Many of the OTC medications you'd normally take to manage symptoms are off-limits (ibuprofen ranks on that list). Staying well is especially crucial during the first trimester, when the fetus's organ systems are developing. High fevers can cause a variety of problems, so wash your hands frequently and have your partner do the same. Speak to a provider about your medication options if you do come down with anything so they can help you manage symptoms.

I already have a germ factory, I mean toddler, at home, and heard about CMV. What is it, and how can I avoid it?

If an existing child attends school or day care, or you work in one, you know that it is impossible to avoid every single circulating virus. However, the one you should take pains to avoid is cytomegalovirus, or CMV. Although it does not impact most babies, it is the leading infectious cause of birth defects, as one in two hundred babies is born with it. The problems CMV causes include hearing and vision loss, microcephaly, seizures, and developmental delays, and, in some rare but severe cases, pregnancy loss. Saliva and urine are the two main transmission vectors, so during pregnancy do not share food, utensils, or cups with any kids under five, and wash your hands the full twenty seconds with soap and water after changing a diaper or helping during toilet time. Better yet, ask your partner to take over butt wiping.

I struggled with infertility and am really anxious. Is that normal?

Anxiety is common during pregnancy no matter what you went through to conceive. It's all new, your body is changing in bizarre and interesting ways, and you are responsible for another life. For some people anxiety comes in waves, and others experience occasional flares. If you are naturally anxious, it may get worse during pregnancy, too.

Many fertility clinics now offer access to mental health services, as anxiety is especially common for infertility patients, and many cite high levels during pregnancy and later as parents. Infertility treatments themselves are traumatic events for many patients, and the loss of control and expectations—which can be years in the making—does not go away overnight (or at all). The uncertainty of early pregnancy can be especially fraught if you've suffered a pregnancy loss. While you may not feel like you have time to explore these feelings during an ob visit, find a trusted person—whether a therapist, nurse, midwife, doula, another complementary provider, or friend who's been through it, too—and open up.

My job involves a lot of travel. Any tips for flying while pregnant?

How much you enjoy getting on a plane will depend on how things are going. Generally, travel in the first trimester is tolerable but not very fun, best in the second (also the time for a babymoon), and increasingly uncomfortable in the third.

Most commercial airlines in the US restrict travel after thirty-six weeks, and international trips can require a doctor's note as early as twenty-eight weeks. Check with your favorite carrier for their specific rules. Do the math on your departure *and* return dates. In addition to that trusty note, it's a good idea to have access to your medical records just in case you have issues while away from home. You can go through the airport security line normally throughout pregnancy. Metal detectors are fine, and though they look dangerous, so are the large body scanners. If you feel safer opting out, step out of line and ask for a physical check.

To optimize your comfort, book an exit row or bulkhead seat to get a few extra inches to stretch out, and slide the seat belt under your belly before you cinch. It's easy to get dehydrated while you're pregnant even when not at thirty thousand feet, so drink plenty of water to combat the plane's low humidity. Wear compression socks, get up, and stretch frequently to reduce the small risk of deep vein thrombosis (DVT), especially if you've had previous clotting issues or are overweight. Drawing the alphabet with your toes every hour helps to keep things moving if you're not on the aisle and are sick of climbing over your neighbor. And instead of loading up with a big meal before you board, especially with foods that cause gas, like cruciferous vegetables and carbonated drinks, try smaller portions and avoid salty foods.

Though I was fine to fly at twenty-seven weeks, I almost did not make it home from London at twenty-nine as I did not have a doctor's note. So please, do the math on your return date and check the airline's policies—especially for international travel.

YOUR CARE TEAM
FANTASY DRAFT

Recruiting the perfect practitioners
to manage your pregnancy

Pregnancy and childbirth used to be community events. Women received advice and help from female friends and family during labor. Men were not part of childbirth; in fact, there were laws in some places that forbade their involvement, as it was considered scandalous even in a healthcare context for any man other than a woman's husband to see her in a state of undress. It wasn't until the 1970s that fathers were widely admitted to the delivery room at all.

Midwives led nearly all pregnancy care and were held in high social regard. But around the time the ink was drying on the Constitution in 1787, American medical schools began to provide formalized obstetric education for physicians. This training was offered only to men, so the primarily female midwives of the age missed out, and male midwives, or the first obstetricians, replaced them.

The shift away from midwifery solidified after Dr. Joseph DeLee, the founder of modern obstetrics, started the Chicago Lying-In Hospital in 1917. His improvement of hygienic practices and medicalized approach to childbirth yielded a maternal mortality rate 25 percent of the national average, which was significant, considering around one in every 154 women at that time died during birth. His innovations included the first portable incubator and fetoscope, and separate facilities and laundry for birthing as preventive measures against hospital-acquired infection, which was a leading cause of maternal death.

While his improvements saved lives and formed the foundation for many of today's medical practices, DeLee's interventionist approach had less-positive effects on pregnancy care, too. One of his legacies was the use of forceps and episiotomy (an incision made in the perineum to enlarge the vaginal opening during childbirth), even when there were no complications that required mechanical intervention. Forty percent of babies born vaginally in the US in the early 1970s were delivered with forceps, and 90 percent of mothers received an episiotomy. Thankfully, research proved that these practices should be exercised only if medically indicated; the episiotomy rate dropped to below 20 percent by 2000 and continues to decline.

Today we're seeing a move back to less intervention and the reemergence of midwives as part of a coordinated care team across all birth settings. Midwives increasingly participate alongside doctors at hospitals and lead nearly all birth center and home births. The out-of-hospital birth rate still hovers between 1 and 2 percent, and the reason they are not more common is risk.

Around one-third of all first-time mothers who attempt home births transfer to the hospital, and babies die at twice the rate during home births as they do in hospitals. The admission rate drops to 9 percent for those who have given birth before, making it a better option for subsequent pregnancies. Home births are intimate, and you'll hear words like *sublime* and *transcendental* used by those who successfully pull one off. But they are appropriate only in low-risk pregnancies.

To be classified as low risk, you must be pregnant with a single baby (no multiples) that is head-down (not breech or sideways), and not have any medical complications like hypertension or diabetes or had prior C-sections (there is an increased risk of uterine rupture). If placental complications like placenta previa or accreta or fetal growth restriction or macrosomia develop during your pregnancy, you will be classified as high risk. Home births must involve experienced practitioners trained in neonatal resuscitation, and ideally, they take place within a fifteen-minute drive of a hospital just in case. The proximity matters because research shows that for emergency deliveries, lowering the decision-to-incision time for a C-section to under thirty minutes significantly improves fetal outcomes. If your baby is having difficulty breathing, less transport time could save its life. If you're considering a home birth, discuss your options with your ob-gyn or midwife, carefully go through the risks, and coordinate a plan.

No matter who you work with, however, standard prenatal visits cannot cover everything. Maintaining a strong pelvic floor, understanding nutrition and exercise, and managing mental health issues are a few examples of important areas that will not be addressed in a normal visit, so ask for referrals to see complementary practitioners. If the idea of scheduling anything other than prenatal appointments feels like too much, have no fear. Telemedicine puts these practices within reach no matter how busy you are or where you live and reduces their costs. Some of the practitioners won't be relevant until later in your pregnancy. But it's helpful to understand how and when they provide value, get a list of referrals early, and factor any additional costs (if they aren't covered) into your budget.

PRENATAL CARE PROVIDERS

The first specialist to draft is the quarterback for your prenatal care. The two most common options are ob-gyns and midwives. If you have a high-risk pregnancy, or are managing a chronic condition (like hypertension or diabetes), starting with an ob-gyn is standard, though you may be able to transition to a midwife if everything progresses drama-free. If your pregnancy is sans complications, a midwife can be the main point of contact during most of your prenatal care. This goes for planned home births and those taking place in birthing centers and, increasingly, in hospital settings. A growing number of hospitals now have midwives on staff and present during birth, regardless of who manages your prenatal care.

If you don't already work with a practitioner you like or have a referral from a friend, start by thinking about your ideal birth experience. For example, if you want to deliver at a birth center, you'll need to find a facility and a practitioner, likely a midwife, approved to practice at said facility. If you have a specific hospital in mind, ensure that your ob-gyn has rights to practice there. A data point to explore if you have several hospital options is the cesarean section rate, as it can vary widely. Next up: Call your insurance provider to see what and whom they cover and see if they have an out-of-pocket estimate. Home births and birth centers are rarely covered by insurance, so if you're a good candidate, you'll likely be on the hook for all of those costs.

Ob-gyns

Most prenatal care and births are led or assisted by an obstetrician-gynecologist. The term *obstetrics* refers to childbirth, and *gynecology* deals with the reproductive health conditions specific to women and girls. Some providers practice both fields, but fun fact: just like all toads are frogs, but not all frogs are toads, not all gynecologists are obstetricians, but all obstetricians are gynecologists. If your provider lacks the "ob" in front of the "gyn," it's time to find someone who doesn't.

Maternal-fetal medicine specialists (MFMs), or, as they're also known, perinatologists, are a subset of ob-gyns that specialize in high-risk pregnancies. Those deemed high-risk may have a consult with an MFM, comanage their care with an ob-gyn and MFM, or just see an MFM for milestones like ultrasounds or exclusively if complications arise.

An ob-gyn's practice can be in an office or a hospital. Specialists in these practices include not only the ob-gyns themselves, but often nurse practitioners, midwives, sonographers, dietitians, genetic counselors, social workers, lactation consultants, and physician assistants.

Your exposure to each subspecialty will depend on the specifics of your pregnancy and your desire to enlist additional help.

Choosing the right ob-gyn is important, as they will be your Sherpa through this long, often confusing, very personal process. However, it's helpful to remember two critical facts about this relationship.

Fact #1: Though you will see this person with increasing frequency toward the end of your pregnancy, your total time together amounts to only a handful of hours, especially if you are low risk. You'll see your provider once per month in the first and second trimesters, once every two weeks in the third trimester up to thirty-six weeks, and once per week from thirty-six weeks through pop time.

Fact #2: A few private practitioners still attend each of their patients' births, especially in rural areas. But in general, the days of ob-gyns on call every night are over. There are high burnout rates associated with the stress of the job, so it's a good thing for patient care that your ob-gyn is rested. Practically speaking, it's unlikely the doctor you've poured out every concern and ache and pain to during prenatal visits will be the one to deliver your baby. If you have strong feelings about this detail, ask about the practice's care model before or during your first prenatal visit to ensure your expectations match their policies. Setting appointments throughout your pregnancy with different ob-gyns to get to know everyone in the practice is a tactic to increase the odds of a friendly face at birth.

Babies show up when they're ready, schedules change, and many hospitals now employ an OB hospitalist model powered by ob-gyns who only practice in the hospital. Think of them as a hospital's commitment to safety, as they are focused solely on childbirth and obstetrical emergencies. They work only in the hospital and do not provide prenatal care, so your odds of seeing them before birth are slim.

Standard prenatal appointment schedule

When	What happens
8–10 weeks	First appointment and ultrasound (you'll also learn your due date, which is really just an estimate!)
10–12 weeks	Initial blood draw for first health screening and noninvasive prenatal testing (NIPS) if requested
12 weeks	Nuchal translucency measurement ultrasound and genetic counseling (if NIPS testing was requested)
16 weeks	Blood tests and prenatal checkup
18–20 weeks	Anatomy scan ultrasound (you'll learn gender if you don't already know!) and prenatal checkup
24 weeks	Glucose screening for gestational diabetes and prenatal check-in
28 weeks	Prenatal check-in
32 weeks	Final ultrasound (typically only done in higher-risk pregnancies) and prenatal check-in
36 weeks	Prenatal check-in
38 weeks	Prenatal check-in
39 weeks	Prenatal check-in
40 weeks	Prenatal check-in

| 41 weeks | Induction of labor if it hasn't started on its own (this can vary by provider and your pregnancy) |
| 1–6 weeks postpartum | If you had high blood pressure during pregnancy, you'll need a checkup within a week of leaving the hospital. Otherwise, your follow-up appointment will happen at six weeks postpartum. |

Each prenatal appointment will include a Q&A session for you, a weight measurement and blood pressure reading, a discussion of new medications or issues since the previous appointment, a chance to listen to your baby's heartbeat, a measurement of your belly (from the second trimester the fundal height, or distance in centimeters from the pubic bone to the top of the uterus, tracks to the number of weeks you are pregnant), a mental health check-in, and any additional tests.

There is also a physical exam, which can include a pelvic exam to check on your internal organs. Pregnancy and childbirth can be difficult for survivors of sexual abuse, and this exam is especially triggering. If this is you, tell your ob-gyn at the beginning of your pregnancy journey so it is noted in your chart. No matter what your history, during a physical exam your provider should always tell you what they're doing before they do it and ask for permission before touching you. If you'd like a chaperone present if your partner or a friend is not there, that's your right, too.

During an appointment, it can be hard to feel like you get all your questions answered, since appointments are ten to fifteen minutes long on average. If you don't understand something your provider said, ask again. Many have visual aids or can draw a picture if that's your learning style. Take notes or enlist your partner to do so.

Afterward, if things come up, you can submit questions via the nurse line, or some providers offer secure messaging through their practice's patient portal.

Some practices are integrating more virtual appointments into this schedule for those with low-risk pregnancies. While chatting from home or work is far more convenient, especially for working parents or those with existing kids, if you'd rather see someone in person, you can request to do so or build relationships with other providers in the practice if yours is not available.

If you need to find someone new, asking for a referral from your primary care provider, friend, colleague, or someone else you trust is a good place to start. Here are a few questions to consider before and during that first appointment:

- Are they in-network for my healthcare coverage?
- What is their hospital affiliation, and where would I deliver?
- If my physician isn't the one to deliver, who will be?
- How does my doctor feel about my birth and pain medication preferences?
- Does the doctor have a good bedside manner?
- What is the makeup of the rest of the practice?
- If your doctor is in a solo practice, who covers when they are not available?
- How can I get in touch during business hours? What about after hours and in case of emergency?
- What is their C-section rate and episiotomy rate, and do they perform VBACs? (VBAC = vaginal birth after C-section)

As a member of the dreaded advanced-maternal-age crew, I was in the high-risk category. This meant I saw an MFM for my pre- natal care. It was unlikely I would see her in the delivery room, so after I passed twenty weeks and was deemed less risky, I booked appointments with other ob-gyns in the practice. All of them had slightly different styles, and I learned a lot seeing a wide range of people.

I knew in advance that this is how things work, so I did not feel any attachment to who was present when I gave birth, though it made having a doula feel doubly important. And I was glad I made my peace with it, as a midwife and an L&D (labor and delivery) nurse started the process, but later an OB hospitalist joined the team, assisted by residents I'd never set eyes on before.

Midwives

Midwives are the primary childbirth providers in most countries around the world, but they attend just 8 percent of US births. Many people assume that midwives, long marked as grandmas in the woods, serve only at home births and do not have formal medical training. While some are based in birthing centers and, yes, supervise home births, a growing number are hospital-based and work alongside ob-gyns. They can manage care throughout pregnancy, birth, and postpartum, primarily in low-risk pregnancies, though they can manage more complicated births under ob-gyn supervision.

The benefits of midwifery's reintegration back into the healthcare system go deep. Hospital births supervised by midwives are less likely to end in a C-section or other medical intervention, and the high-touch model can be much more emotionally fulfilling. Individuals cared for by midwives cite a better experience and higher levels of autonomy before and after childbirth, especially when care is delivered in community settings instead of hospitals.

Outside of medical training, the biggest difference in care between an ob-gyn and a midwife is the appointment experience. Ob-gyn visits are focused on tests, metrics, and clinical care. Midwives spend more time with patients, focus less on interventions and more on unmedicated options before and during birth, and cater to the emotional side of pregnancy. Like ob-gyn practices, most hospital-based midwifery practices also operate in a cohort model, which means you may see a variety of practitioners during your pregnancy and that it's not always possible to guarantee who will be at your birth.

There are several certification levels for midwives, and which type you'll find is a function of your geography and desired birth setting. The main differences are the type of training they receive and whether they have a nursing certification. **Certified nurse-midwives (CNMs)** are found in more traditional medical settings, as they are licensed registered nurses who go on to earn a midwifery certification. Some CNMs perform home births and practice at birthing centers, but the majority work alongside ob-gyns in private or hospital settings. They can provide the full spectrum of prenatal care, and most can write prescriptions. **Certified midwives (CMs)** take the same exam as CNMs, and though their graduate-level education and testing are the same as CNMs, they do not have a nursing degree. **Certified professional midwives (CPMs)** are most often present at home births or in birth centers, and their training requires experience in both. Training is less standardized than for CMs and CNMs, and they are generally not licensed nurses.

There can be challenges to working with a midwife. The first: geographical rules that dictate the limits of their practice, and whether they are allowed to practice at all. (Ironically, the states with the most restrictive policies also have the highest rates of adverse birth outcomes!) While rules are changing, there can also be issues paying for midwives, as private insurance often lacks in-network providers or refuses to cover their services at all.

While I did not manage my prenatal care with a midwife, there was one at my son's birth. She was a white-haired oasis of calm and made such an impression that even now many years later she makes cameos in my dreams.

Family practice physicians

If you already see someone you love for everyday issues and are low risk, it's fine to start prenatal care with your family-practice physician. The main benefit is they already know you and your medical history and can later take on the role of pediatrician when your baby comes along.

However, their training is focused on a range of medical conditions, not obstetrics, so few are equipped to handle high-risk pregnancies. If you run into complications, they will refer you to an ob-gyn, and may not be the one to handle labor and delivery.

Group prenatal care

Many hospitals and private medical practices offer group prenatal care, which brings together pregnant women due around the same time. You'll still have a one-on-one relationship with an ob-gyn or midwife, but care is not constrained to short individual exams. Instead, each session is about sixty to ninety minutes and includes your prenatal appointment and a group discussion. Studies have shown improved pregnancy outcomes with this model.

Another benefit is making friends who are in exactly the same life stage. Some families even stage reunions, or pool childcare resources. Like working with a midwife, group care is generally utilized in low-risk pregnancies, though it's possible to take advantage of both individual appointments and a group setting if you are high-risk and want the additional support.

Doulas

Translated from Greek, the word *doula* literally means "woman's servant." Doulas are health professionals who provide emotional, physical, and educational support to you and your partner before, during, and after birth. This support ranges from knowing when it's time to go to the hospital and coaching you (and your partner) through birth, to help with breastfeeding and recovery afterward. They cannot prescribe drugs, diagnose health conditions, or perform clinical procedures, as very few have medical backgrounds. You can think of them as standing in for the village that used to surround birthing women.

There are many high-quality studies cited in this book's bibliography touting the benefits of doulas. Here are a few: Women with continuous support during labor are more likely to have spontaneous vaginal births and shorter labor. They are also less likely to have C-sections and need less pain medication. Their babies have higher Apgar scores (the test done right after birth to quickly summarize a newborn's health) and less trouble breastfeeding and caring for their infants. In general, everyone also leaves the birth experience feeling more positive. Right now, doulas are only present at around 6 percent of births, but the number of providers is growing, and public awareness of these benefits is increasing.

So how is it doulas are so effective? Well, labor can be long, especially in a first birth, and if it is, there may be stretches of time when you and your partner are left alone. Labor and delivery nurses are amazing, but they have more than one patient, and their priority is to provide clinical care. Same for midwives and ob-gyns. It's helpful to have someone around who has seen a few births to remind you that yes, the baby will come out eventually, and cheer you on. Doulas are not hospital employees—they are there just for you. And they are just as valuable to your partner (in some cases even more so), even if only to give them an occasional break.

Some doulas have strong opinions about the use of interventions, C-sections, and the appropriate scope of medical care, so understanding their birth philosophy is important. Their role is not to tell you how to give birth, or to overrule your physician; it's to determine your values, provide information, and answer questions, then support you in whatever birthing process you choose. If you're giving birth at a hospital, let your physician know you're planning to hire a doula at a prenatal appointment so they can note it in your chart. There can be tension between medical professionals and doulas, which is best relieved through open communication and mutual respect.

The time to start looking for a doula is at the beginning of the second trimester, as many of them book up far in advance. The official start of your doula relationship is at the beginning of the third trimester and lasts through the first weeks postpartum. Pre-birth meetings focus on understanding your needs, creating birth preferences, and teaching your partner how to be part of the labor process. Many doulas are also childbirth educators; in fact, some lead the classes taught at hospitals. When it comes time for birth, they will be on call during early labor, then join you at home until it's go time. During active labor, they will help you relax, practice nonmedical pain relief techniques, and be your advocate if needed. After your baby arrives, most doulas hang around to help with breastfeeding, and visit after you return home. Some even provide ongoing support through the first year of your infant's life.

A referral from a friend or healthcare provider or fitness studio that teaches prenatal classes is another great way to find a doula. If you're starting cold, Dona.org, the largest credentialing organization for doulas, has a database of their certified practitioners to search. Interview several to see what style and approach is right for you, and include your partner in these discussions, since they will spend just as much time with the doula as you will. While certification and experience are important, just as critical are trust and whether you feel at ease in their company. Things get intimate during birth (perineal heating pads, anyone?), so be comfortable with the idea of your doula touching and coaching you during the intensity of labor.

Here are a few questions to ask during the doula interview process:

- Where did you receive your labor support training? Do you have any additional certifications or training?
- How long have you been practicing and how many births have you attended?

- What are your values and goals in providing your services to families?
- What is your approach to interactions with a medical team? Do you typically practice in hospitals?
- How do you handle long births? Do you leave to sleep/ take breaks?
- What kind of support do you provide for partners?
- Can you share an outline of the visits we'll have before and after birth?
- How many clients do you take each month?
- What happens when I go into labor? What kind of support do you provide?
- What if labor happens before or after my due date and you are not available? Do you work in a team? How many times have you needed a backup doula?
- What are your fees and what is included?

Now, the bad news. Even though there is a compelling financial case for doulas to be present at every single birth (like the 41 percent reduction in C-section rates), it's still rare that insurance or Medicaid will pay. Employers that offer pregnancy benefits allow reimbursement, and if you're paying out of pocket, some doulas operate on a sliding scale, while others have fixed rates. But any way you cut it, having a doula at your birth—even if it requires trimming back in other areas or registering for one as a baby shower gift—is an investment worth making.

Hiring a doula—or, in our case, two women who worked as a team—was the best decision I made during pregnancy. They taught our birth class; provided text support, coaching, and hairbrushing during sixty-plus hours of labor; advocated for me when things got complicated; gave my husband, Nick, breaks; performed postpartum check-ins; created an atmosphere of calm; and helped us anticipate what was coming next at every twist and turn.

After personal experience and the huge glut of research demonstrating improved clinical outcomes, I'm pushing everyone I meet—health systems, ob-gyns, politicians and government officials, and insurers—to make doulas a standard part of childbirth for every family.

Therapists

Pregnancy is supposed to be the happiest time of your life, right? Friends and family are excited, and you're sporting a gorgeous pregnant glow and on the cusp of welcoming a brand-new life that *you* created in *your* body from scratch. Isn't that beautiful? How could anyone need therapy at such a perfectly lovely time?

As you've probably figured out by now, the journey to becoming a parent isn't always sunshine and puppies. Sometimes it's *hard*. Even if it's relatively painless, it's a huge personal transformation. Your identity changes. Your hormones change. Your body changes. Your partnership changes. Your friendships change. Your professional life, finances, and responsibilities do, too. Some of these changes are great. Some less so.

Talking to your pumped-up inner circle on the down days can feel off-limits in the face of so much enthusiasm. Which is why having an impartial third party around is so helpful.

Therapy isn't just for when things go wrong. Nor does it have to involve lying on a couch dissecting your relationship with your mother. Or father. Or ex-boyfriend. Therapy is unfairly associated only with people who are unhappy or dealing with a clinical condition when in fact, it's valuable when applied to life transitions and utilized for smaller periods of time, too.

Four in five women report mood changes associated with pregnancy and postpartum, and one in five women report depression or anxiety. Even that number is believed to be wildly underreported. So if you're reading this and thinking, *That's me*, you are not alone. Therapy should be a standard part of pre- and postnatal care and a requirement for anyone who is navigating infertility. Making time to see a therapist may not feel like it fits into your busy life. But good news: They are available by phone, video chat, and text.

Eating my feelings was not an effective coping strategy by pregnancy number three. I'd used therapy previously to get through life transitions, so it felt like a natural solution. A friend supplied a referral to a grief counselor, and I committed to go as many times as needed to work through my unresolved feelings.

Therapy didn't replace my friends or Nick. Despite their support and love, there were things I couldn't say out loud to them. And that's the beautiful thing about therapy—you can say anything and the therapist not only won't tell anyone; they actually can't. Legally! For me, therapy is a safe place to unload those secret, sometimes irrational thoughts in a judgment-free environment, to someone trained to help you make sense of it all.

GETTING THE MOST OUT OF YOUR CARE TEAM

Deciding which providers and practices fit best into your life and align with your values is up to you. Once you assemble your dream team, ensure that you are communicating and making decisions together, and that you share anything important from other appointments.

Another consideration is how you best process information, and what type and amount of data helps you feel confident. For example, if you like to outsource to the experts, you may not care as much about stats and the reasoning behind a care plan. The opposite is true if you are a data driven person who enjoys analyzing every possible option.

No matter where you are on the spectrum, let your providers know so they can calibrate the amount and type of information they provide at appointments.

It's your right to ask as many questions as it takes for you to feel comfortable—no matter how silly they might seem at the time. This can feel awkward if an appointment feels rushed. Pro tip: Keep a list of questions that come up at home on your phone so you can avoid getting into the car after an appointment and thinking, *I wish I'd asked [fill in blank]*.

THINGS TO AVOID

The truth about drugs and alcohol, how to select safe products, and navigating cosmetic procedures

If you haven't experienced it yet, brace yourself. The moment people find out that you are pregnant, a tidal wave of differing opinions—regarding what to eat, how to deal with morning sickness, which baby items you absolutely must have, exercise, and everything else you never asked—will be unleashed.

Perhaps it's the universe preparing you for the glut of unsolicited parenting advice you'll soon receive. Maybe there is something so tantalizing about that cute bump that people can't help but, well, want to be helpful. The point is, everyone, including your neighbors, friends, colleagues, and yes, complete strangers will have different guidance, much of it useless.

To build a baseline for decision-making, let's start by understanding the ins and outs of the posh aquatic habitat your baby is occupying in your abdomen. The uterus and placenta are the two main organs involved in growing a baby. Prepregnancy, the uterus is about the size of a fist; it expands to the size of a watermelon to accommodate your growing baby. The placenta is a miraculous organ grown only during pregnancy that attaches to the wall of your uterus. It serves as the interface between mother and baby, via the umbilical cord. The placenta does many cool things, like let oxygen in and carbon dioxide out, facilitate the transfer of nutrients between you and your baby, and remove the resulting waste. It then exits your body right after birth, as it serves no other function. In any future pregnancy, you'll grow a brand-new placenta.

The placenta can also let in things that are not good for your baby's development. These harmful substances are known as teratogens, and they are a cause of birth defects. A teratogen's ability to cross into the placenta determines how harmful it is, and this ability is why the medical community is so strongly against your ingesting or being around known teratogens like alcohol, recreational drugs, nicotine, and carbon monoxide while you are pregnant.

So when, specifically, during a pregnancy is this crossing most likely to cause issues? The short answer is, it's never a good idea to expose a growing fetus to anything that could cause harm. However, you may hear doctors say that the first trimester is when you should pay the most attention. Here's why.

Though it sounds like a time when dinosaurs roamed the earth, the teratogenic period happens in the forty-day stretch between day thirty-one and day seventy-one after your LMP. In other words, if you have a twenty-eight-day cycle, it starts three days after you've missed your period. You may or may not even know you're pregnant yet. But this stretch is when developing systems have the highest likelihood of being affected, and when many birth defects occur.

The effects vary and are hard to predict. Genetics are a factor, as is the level of exposure. Some babies make it through subjection to recreational or prescribed drugs during a full pregnancy with no adverse effects, and some do not. Two to 3 percent of all pregnancies are affected by issues that occur during this period.

Now that we understand the biological mechanics, let's focus more specifically on the most important teratogens to avoid while pregnant. This includes everything from the obvious, like cigarettes, to the less discussed, like prescription medications and Botox. What follows is a full list of chemicals and the products they are most found in to make swapping to a clean routine easy.

One other note: Product descriptors like *organic* and *natural* across food, cosmetics, and cleaning products have absolutely no legal meaning. While it's easy to assume that these terms mean nothing artificial or synthetic is included as an ingredient, that is not always the case. If using clean products is important to you, read labels carefully and check the consumer guides on the Environmental Working Group's website.

ALCOHOL

Alcohol consumption is perhaps the most hotly debated subject you'll encounter during pregnancy. What's not up for debate is that heavy drinking during pregnancy—more than two drinks per day—can cause birth defects and fetal alcohol syndrome and can lead to behavioral and mental health issues for a child later in life. Alcohol is a known teratogen, and the number of children affected by fetal alcohol syndrome spectrum disorders today is higher than the number diagnosed with autism.

What's less clear is the impact of more casual, moderate drinking— one to two drinks per day or less. Studies show that even small amounts of alcohol can cause behavioral problems, though there are so many confounding factors related to parenting styles, psychographic factors, use of other substances, and environment that it's hard to know if alcohol was the root cause.

I know, I know. Your grandparents drank while pregnant and your parents are fine. Maybe your mom did and you're okay, too. European women don't give up wine. (Or do they?) This topic also feels like yet another area where "better safe than sorry" is the best rationale we have, and this is more about our willingness to trust women to exercise self-control. Your taste buds change along with your sense of smell when you become pregnant, and some women report an aversion to alcohol as an early symptom, citing a bitter taste. This distaste can persist throughout pregnancy, so it may be that alcohol is no longer appealing anyway.

On the point of self-control, unless you want to haul a hydrometer or alcohol meter around, it's impossible to know exactly how much alcohol makes it into your system, as beers and spirits have different proofs from label to label, and bartenders don't always pour consistent amounts. This issue of volume and alcohol content per serving is one reason that guidelines are and will remain conservative regardless of your willingness to self-police.

Let's get back to the science. If you rely on research to reveal a definitive answer as to whether light or moderate drinking is okay, sorry to say there isn't one. If you'd like to find research open-ended enough to justify continuing to drink, there are studies that show light use has no known risks. However, a major flaw of these studies is that they rely on self-reported data, which means the only input is the subjects' memories and their understanding of how many drinks they consumed. And in the words of the researchers who performed these studies, no evidence of harm is not the same as evidence of no harm.

As you have already heard a thousand times, complete abstinence is what all medical professionals and organizations recommend throughout pregnancy, simply because we do not understand the long-term implications. Nor are we likely to anytime soon, due to the lack of large, randomized, controlled studies, reliance on less rigorous research methods, and underlying ethical dilemmas of doing this research in the first place.

European countries are conservative with their recommendations too. France advocates 100 percent abstinence during pregnancy, the UK changed its guidance from abstaining during conception and the first trimester to the entirety of pregnancy, and Italy warns its pregnant mothers against the possible side effects of alcohol, too.

Alcohol consumption is declining anyway, and a growing number of tasty mocktails, shrubs, and nonalcoholic beers are available on most menus. If you feel self-conscious at happy hour in the early months before you're showing, there are strategies until your news is more public. Any bartender or server will be game to help you out, so if not drinking seems tantamount to spilling the beans, get to the bar or restaurant early to place an order. Drinks like "vodka soda" (hold the vodka) or a sparkling beverage with a citrus or herb garnish are convincing fakes. And remember, just the act of holding something in your hand will be enough to avert most suspicion.

Though it may seem overly conservative, in the scheme of things you sacrifice while pregnant (your body, your sleep, your ability to form coherent sentences), booze is a pretty small one.

> *I thought giving up alcohol would be a struggle, as I used to really enjoy wine. Surprise, surprise—I found the smell and tiny sips of all forms of alcohol gross and vinegar-like from the early days until I gave birth. Though I like having a cocktail now and then, pregnancy may have rewired my taste buds permanently, as my interest in alcohol now is somewhere between occasional and zero.*

SMOKING AND VAPING

This is an easy one, as the research is very clear: Smoking, whether it's cigarettes, cigars, vaping, or cigarillos, should not be done at all during pregnancy or while trying to conceive. Smoking makes it harder to get pregnant and stay pregnant, can cause premature birth or birth defects like a cleft palate, and, after pregnancy, is a risk factor for sudden infant death syndrome (SIDS). Secondhand smoke is also harmful, so to reduce exposure stay out of enclosed smoky spaces and ask your partner to quit, too.

Though e-cigarettes don't come packed with the same myriad of harmful chemicals as traditional cigarettes, nicotine can still cause issues with your baby's lungs and brain. In other words, any nicotine delivery system is off-limits while you're pregnant.

CANNABIS AND RECREATIONAL DRUGS

Using any recreational drugs, from MDMA to cocaine and fentanyl or hallucinogens, during pregnancy is a hard no.

A drug many people still question, however, is cannabis because it comes from a plant. (So does cocaine, by the way.) Over 180 million people around the world use some form of cannabis, and it is available as a supplement in drinks, food, and cosmetics. Though there are eighty-five different types of cannabinoids, we'll focus on the two most popular: tetrahydrocannabinol (THC) and cannabidiol (CBD).

THC is derived from marijuana and is still illegal in many places around the world, though it's legal in much of the US. While it has proven health benefits, like helping with the side effects of cancer treatment, it also causes the euphoric feeling known as getting high.

CBD is primarily derived from hemp and, because it lives in a grayer legal area, is widely available. CBD delivers many of the same health benefits of THC but is growing in popularity because it does so without the high. Found in everything from infused coffee and cocktails to facial creams, it's used to help with pain and stress relief. Though THC and CBD are biologically almost identical, one atomic-level difference is responsible for their divergent effects in the body.

So why the pharmacology lesson? The Drug Enforcement Agency (DEA) requires a license to run trials involving cannabis, and limits where the strains can be sourced. Add to that the questionable ethics of testing substances on pregnant women and babies, and, as with alcohol and prescription medications, you have a paucity of solid data.

Here is what we know: THC produces genetic changes in sperm and affects the pathway that helps bodily organs grow to full size as well as the genes that regulate growth during development. It's not yet known whether these changes are passed down to the child. Maternal THC use has been linked to low birth weights and a higher

likelihood of placement in the NICU for babies, as well as to anemia in the mothers. So recreational use of THC—and even secondhand exposure to it—is a bad idea while you are pregnant or trying
to conceive.

The research on CBD is less clear because it has not been studied as extensively. An FDA-approved CBD-powered pharmaceutical
called Epidiolex gives us the best information to date on the safety of
CBD for pregnant and lactating women based on two animal studies
with rabbits and rats. They concluded that negative outcomes happened at 125 milligrams per kilogram, which for a 150-pound woman
is 8,500 milligrams—much higher than the 10 milligrams per serving
found in the commonly available tinctures and infused drinks. Doses
of almost anything at that level, even prenatal vitamins, can be harmful, so it's not surprising.

More problematic if you do want to use CBD-powered products: A
labeling accuracy study done by the FDA reported that only twenty-six
of eighty-four CBD products contained the amount claimed; eighteen
of them contained THC, and enough of it to cause intoxication or
impairment. So even if you think a product is safe to use, due to the
Wild West regulatory environment and lack of rigorous product testing, there are no guarantees.

Some practitioners are exploring CBD as an alternative treatment
for conditions like postpartum psychosis, as it may be more effective
and safer than prescription medications. If it is presented as a clinical
treatment option and you want to confirm what you're taking is of high
quality, there are a few easy steps:

- Ask the company for a certificate of analysis (COA)
  done by an objective, third-party lab.
- Match the milligrams of CBD (and any other
  cannabinoids) per serving to the label's claim.
- Make sure the COA includes comprehensive testing for
  pesticides, molds, chemicals, and solvents—and shows
  they are not detected.

- The COA should be lot specific, and your product should match.

However, let it be repeated that using these products outside of medical supervision while trying to conceive, pregnant, or breastfeeding is not advisable, so always seek a professional's help.

COSMETIC PROCEDURES

Procedure	Advice
Injectables (fillers, Botox/ neuromodulators)	No, wait until finished with breastfeeding
Laser hair removal/ sclerotherapy	No, wait until finished with breastfeeding
Tattoos/piercings	No, wait until finished with breastfeeding
Facials	Yes, though check ingredients
Hair treatments	Yes, though consider waiting until after the first trimester and always receive treatments in well-ventilated spaces
Manicures/ pedicures	Yes, though skip the gel polish, receive treatments in well-ventilated spaces, and ensure the salon practices safe hygiene methods and uses sterilized tools

If you are a fan of Botox (a.k.a. neuromodulators) and fillers and facials and laser hair removal, I have good news and bad news. Well, actually, it's mostly bad news. As with cannabinoids, the ethics of testing elective cosmetic procedures on pregnant women and babies are . . . questionable, which means the number of human studies conducted is low. Frustrating, I know.

Injectables

The main issue is whether injectable and topical compounds can cross the placental barrier to the baby. Botulinum toxin, the main ingredient in Botox, has a heavy molecular weight that makes it unlikely to do so, but in FDA animal studies high doses were shown to cause low birth weight, skeletal ossification, miscarriage, premature delivery, maternal toxicity, and even death. There are no clinical studies that involve pregnant humans. The same goes for lactating humans, where the concern is absorption and incorporation of these products into breast milk.

If you read the labels, product manufacturers consistently state that fillers and neuromodulators are not for use by pregnant or lactating women. Allergan, the manufacturer of Botox, claims it should be used only "if the potential benefit justifies the potential risk to the fetus," thus putting the responsibility back on the medical provider. Even without those warnings, most medical spas and physicians will not perform elective cosmetic procedures involving these products on pregnant or lactating women due to the lack of conclusive data. Too much liability. If you use Botox for a medical condition, your physician will help you weigh the pros and cons of continuing its use.

Laser hair removal and sclerotherapy

So what about laser hair removal (epilation) and sclerotherapy for those pesky pregnancy varicose veins? Both are best kept for your post-pregnancy life, as varicose veins often clear up on their own, and there is a somewhat theoretical (but real) concern around epilation because amniotic fluid may conduct galvanic current. Not to mention any hair you lasered off before pregnancy may sprout up again during those nine months and again later during a future pregnancy.

Tattoos and piercings

Thinking of getting inked to commemorate your new addition? Tattoos and piercings should wait until after birth. This category also includes procedures like microblading, or any others which inject dye into the skin. The main concern is contracting an infection like hepatitis B or HIV from exposure to contaminated needles, but there is also a lack of solid research on the effects of skin dyes, especially during those critical first twelve weeks.

Facials

Now, some good news! Even though you may already be sporting a rosy glow, there are plenty of ways to get safe facials. If you like chemical peels, they are primarily done with glycolic acid, lactic acid, salicylic acid, Jessner solution, and trichloroacetic acid (TCA). Of these, glycolic and lactic acid masks and peels are considered safe because their dermal penetration is negligible.

With the slew of facial products available these days, you should have no problem working out a solution with your aesthetician. Communicate clearly about your pregnancy, ingredients you'd like to avoid, and any concerns, and they will find a way to help you feel and look great.

Hair treatments

More good news: Most hair treatments are considered fine, too. Research is limited when it comes to hair dyes, but the majority are nontoxic and only a small amount is absorbed into the skin. The same is true while you are breastfeeding, as dye does not enter your bloodstream.

There are many vegetable-based and low-ammonia options available. If you'd like to play it safe, substitute highlights for full color, as the dye during highlighting is applied only to your hair, not your scalp. Many physicians suggest waiting until after the first trimester to do any treatments as an extra precaution, and to do it in a well-ventilated area with gloves if you are applying it at home. One important note on hair: Its texture, fullness, and oil content change during pregnancy (also afterward), so your normal products and treatments may not have the same effects you're used to.

Manicures and pedicures

Changes in your nails are another side effect of increased hormones. Some people's nails grow more quickly and are hard as a rock; others become brittle and split easily.

If you like to manage stress in a massage chair surrounded by celebrity gossip magazines while someone goes ham on your cuticles, you can continue as usual during pregnancy—with one change. To you long-lasting-polish lovers, gel is not recommended for a few reasons. Most gel polishes include methyl methacrylate monomer, which can cause allergic reactions, and the twenty-minute acetone soak to remove them has not been studied enough for the risks to be fully understood. As with any cosmetic treatment, tell your technician you are pregnant so they can exercise extra caution.

Otherwise, the rules are the same as those you'd follow while not pregnant. Any salon you visit should be well ventilated and employ safe hygiene practices, like sterilizing and cleaning tools, and have a clear health inspection record. The same goes for at-home manis and pedis: Do it in a room with good ventilation, clean your implements, and skip the gel.

Personal care products and makeup

The beauty and cosmetics industry is notoriously unregulated in the United States, so don't expect any of your products to be labeled as not for pregnant women even if they contain the ingredients listed later in this section. There are many "natural" products that have been shown to adversely affect pregnancy and fetal development, so here's another reminder to check the labels.

Your skin is your body's biggest organ, and a few topical treatments like salicylic acid and retinoids have been shown to cause birth defects. When you review the top ingredients to avoid, where they are most commonly found, how they are labeled, and their side effects, you may question using them even after pregnancy.

Ingredients to avoid

Ingredient	What is it?	Labeled as
Retinoids	Ingredient in prescription acne and antiaging medications	Retinoic acid, retinyl palmitate, retinaldehyde, adapalene, tretinoin, tazarotene, and isotretinoin
	Risk factors	
	There's a proven link between the use of retinoids and an increased risk of birth defects for developing babies. Stop taking them several months before you plan to get pregnant.	
Hydroquinone	A skin-lightening agent used to treat conditions such as chloasma and melasma	Hydroquinone, idrochinone, and quinol/1-4 dihydroxybenzene/1-4 hydroxybenzene
	Risk factors	
	As much as 45 percent of this medication is absorbed into the skin, and while no studies have yet been conducted on the effect of hydroquinone on a fetus, there is just too much of the chemical in your bloodstream after use to justify the risk.	

Ingredient	What is it?	Labeled as
Phthalates	Chemicals added to plastics to make them more flexible and to increase the strength and effectiveness of other chemicals, such as perfume or nail polish	BzBP, DBP, DEP, DMP, or diethyl, dibutyl, or benzylbutyl phthalate

Risk factors

Linked to everything from high blood pressure to ADHD to diabetes. New studies found connections between prenatal phthalate exposure and abnormal fetal development. Look for personal care products that are labeled "phthalate-free."

Formaldehyde	A known carcinogen found in personal care products, including hair-straightening treatments, nail polish, and eyelash glue	Formaldehyde, quaternium-15, dimethyl-dimethyl (DMDM), hydantoin, imidazolidinyl urea, diazolidinyl urea, sodium hydroxymethylglycinate, and 2-bromo-2-nitropropane-1,3-diol (bronopol)

Risk factors

Exposure is linked to spontaneous abortion, congenital malformations, and premature birth. Stick with nail polishes labeled "3-free" or "5-free," and skip the gel manis and pedis.

Ingredients to avoid (continued)

Ingredient	What is it?	Labeled as
Salicylic acid	Acne, exfoliating products (like combination peels), and cleansers	Salicylic acid

Risk factors

Talk to your practitioner about topical versions, but avoid oral forms, as they can cause intracranial bleeding and other defects in the developing fetus. If you need help with sloughing or skin radiance, use products that include glycolic, lactic, or mandelic acids.

Ingredient	What is it?	Labeled as
Aluminum chloride hexahydrate	Common ingredient in high-powered antiperspirants	Aluminum chloride hexahydrate

Risk factors

A common ingredient in prescription and some OTC antiperspirants, aluminum chloride hexahydrate affects the cells that produce sweat.

Ingredient	What is it?	Labeled as
Chemical sunscreens	Sunscreens that create a chemical reaction and work by changing UV rays into heat, then release that heat from the skin.	Avobenzone, homosalate, octisalate, octocrylene, oxybenzone, octinoxate, menthyl anthranilate, and dihydroxyacetone

Risk factors

Can cause harmful cell changes during embryonic development. Stick to mineral sunscreens and physical blockers powered by zinc oxide and titanium dioxide.

Ingredient	What is it?	Labeled as
Parabens	A common preservative in cosmetics used for its antibacterial and fungicidal properties	Propyl-, butyl, isopropyl, isobutyl, and methyl-paraben

Risk factors

Parabens are known hormone disruptors and are easily absorbed into the skin. Prenatal exposure to BPA (a paraben type) has been linked to pregnancy and childhood issues, including miscarriage, low birth weight, obesity, impaired fetal growth, and behavioral problems.

Ingredient	What is it?	Labeled as
Essential oils	A concentrated hydrophobic liquid containing aroma compounds from plants	If the label includes fragrance oil, nature identical, or perfume oil, they are often synthetic and should be avoided.

Risk factors

Because there are so many types available, it's best to go over the safety of any individual oil with your doctor.

PREGNANT BODIES ARE STRONG BODIES

Nutrition, exercise, and managing aches and pains

Throughout human history, pregnant bodies were hidden from the public eye, and pregnant women are still sometimes referred to as being in a "delicate condition." While rest is crucial after birth, unless your pregnancy is high risk, there is no other time in a woman's life when it is more important to be strong and healthy than during pregnancy. This means following a moderate diet, staying active, and dealing with the inevitable physical issues that arise. It does not mean an ultra-restrictive crash diet, or super-high-intensity workouts.

Sticking to a healthy lifestyle during pregnancy has its challenges. Morning sickness can kill your ability to diversify beyond crackers and dry toast or move off your couch. Cravings may inspire strange pairings like pickles and chocolate cake. Acid reflux can make eating pretty much anything unpleasant. As the weeks and months wear on, meals may need to be smaller and smaller to fit in there at all. With the changes to your body, your normal range of physical activities must change, too. If you're using GLP-agonists to manage a health condition like type-2 diabetes or obesity, you must stop, as early studies show a higher risk of miscarriage and birth defects. And stopping may mean your appetite and cravings change.

Before we dig into nutrition, let's talk about an adage that fuels one of the biggest pregnancy myths: eating for two. The average baby weighs between seven and eight pounds at birth, which is sadly not enough to justify doubling your dietary throughput at any point during pregnancy. The amount of weight your practitioner suggests gaining during pregnancy is tied to your body mass index (BMI). Invented in the 1800s by a Belgian mathematician named Adolphe Quetelet, the index is still the most common way we measure obesity, even though BMI is a terrible way to express a single score of one's health. The calculation does not account for muscular frames (muscle is denser than fat), so athletes are often flagged as overweight. Example: Clocking in at 240 pounds and a height of six foot two, Arnold Schwarzenegger has a BMI of 30.8, qualifying him for the obese category. Tom Cruise is five foot seven and 166 pounds, which makes his BMI 26—overweight. BMI also does not account for *where* a person carries weight. Even for those categorized as "normal," whether it accumulates around the hips, stomach, or butt can indicate increased risk of heart disease and diabetes. For that reason, hip and waist measurements are more accurate.

That helping of BMI haterade aside, it's still how your weight will be evaluated at appointments. Below is the chart they use to make recommendations for singleton (one baby) pregnancies. For twins and multiples, these numbers are slightly higher. Note that this is not a mandate—it's an estimate and should be discussed with your provider.

Prepregnancy weight	Recommended weight gain
Underweight (BMI <18.5)	28 to 40 lbs.
Normal weight (BMI 18.5 to 24.9)	25 to 35 lbs.
Overweight (BMI 25 to 29.9)	15 to 25 lbs.
Obese (BMI 30 or more)	11 to 20 lbs.

When it comes to timing, unless you're underweight, it's not necessary to gain any weight in the first trimester. In fact, some women lose a few pounds thanks to morning sickness. If that's you, don't stress. During the second and third trimesters, the only additional nutritional need is a balanced snack. Weight gain during pregnancy is not linear, so if you're tracking, don't expect to gain the same amount every week. Everyone's body is different, and if there's a reason to worry, your practitioner will let you know. Every practitioner has a slightly different approach to these sticky dynamics. Some will share your weight each time; others will record it without comment. If you don't want to be reminded at every appointment, ask to be told only if there's an issue. If you've struggled with an eating disorder, mention it at an early appointment.

So where does this extra weight go? If you're retaining water, you may think it all goes to your cankles. But here is the real answer:

- **7.5 lbs.** Average full-term baby
- **7 lbs.** Stores of fat and other nutrients
- **8 lbs.** Increased blood and fluid volume
- **2 lbs.** Breasts
- **2 lbs.** Uterus
- **2 lbs.** Amniotic fluid
- **1.5 lbs.** Placenta

You will absolutely gain weight while you are pregnant. You are *supposed* to gain weight while you are pregnant. Eat moderately and do as best you can. Unless there is a medical reason, it's not healthy to weigh yourself every day. Get help if you find yourself obsessing about every single fluctuation and try not to compare your weight gain to friends, celebrities, or photos online.

I tracked my weight once a week solely for the purpose of chiming in here. My weight gain was not linear. I didn't gain any weight in the first trimester, then gained ten pounds in the second and fourteen in the third. Some weeks I gained nothing, some I lost weight, and others I gained two or three pounds. My raging acid reflux started in the first trimester and didn't really go away until after birth, which meant I couldn't eat much at a single sitting. I ate smaller meals and snacks throughout the day with the goal of being moderate, not restrictive. During my pregnancy with my second son, I gained exactly the same amount of weight, even though he arrived three weeks earlier than my first.

WHAT TO EAT

What you eat, your baby eats, too. And eating well helps with their development and health. Knowing that makes it tempting to obsess about every single thing you put in your mouth. However, nine months is a long time and requires a more sustainable approach: paying attention and trying your best. You already know consuming pints of cookies-and-cream with reckless abandon isn't a good idea. Instead of the latest fad diet, going full keto, practicing intermittent fasting, or doing anything else that involves skipping meals or cutting out carbs entirely, try following the 80/20 rule: Eighty percent of your diet is whole, unprocessed foods, and 20 percent is foods that are considered less healthy, which are meant to be enjoyed in moderation. Unless you have specific dietary needs, this approach is more sustainable and can last through an entire pregnancy without making you feel deprived.

So what makes a good pregnancy diet? It isn't that different from eating well when you are not pregnant: a mix of lean proteins, whole grains, dairy, and fruits and vegetables (please wash them well!) that come from the produce section instead of boxes and bags.

Pregnancy power foods

Proteins

- **Eggs**—choline, iron, and folate
- **Fish** (oily fish like salmon are ideal)—omega-3 fatty acids (DHA and EPA), B vitamins, potassium, and protein
- **Lean beef and pork**—iron and folate
- **Nuts**—fiber, folate, antioxidants, iron, zinc, and potassium
- **Beans and lentils**—iron, folate, zinc, and calcium

Vegetables

- **Dark green and leafy vegetables** (kale, collard greens, spinach, asparagus, and broccoli)—antioxidants, calcium, folate, vitamin A, potassium, and fiber
- **Sweet potatoes**—packed with fiber and vitamins B6 and C, iron, potassium, and beta-carotene

Fruits

- **Avocado**—fatty acids, fiber, potassium, copper, and vitamins C, E, and K
- **Berries**—antioxidants, fiber, and vitamin C
- **Oranges**—folate and vitamin C
- **Mangoes**—fiber and vitamins A and C
- **Pears**—folate, fiber, and potassium
- **Pomegranates**—folate, iron, protein, fiber, calcium, and vitamin K

Whole grains

- Oatmeal—protein, fiber, and vitamin B6
- **Millet, quinoa, bulgur, and barley**—protein, fiber, antioxidants, magnesium, folate, copper, iron, and manganese
- **Brown or wild rice**—folate, potassium, calcium, manganese, and vitamin B2

Dairy

- **Greek yogurt** (or low-sugar, high-protein alternatives)—calcium, fiber, protein, zinc, and B vitamins
- **Milk** (individually wrapped or sliced cheeses are a solid snack)—calcium, protein, iodine, potassium, and B vitamins

Hate to cook or don't know where to start? There are services that craft delightful, properly portioned meals that arrive on your doorstep ready to eat, or pre-chopped and primed to pop into the oven. Some are even formulated specifically for pregnancy or the postpartum period. If you don't mind a little cooking, make easy-to-reheat meals a few times a week so your fridge is always stocked with things you like. Always carry healthy snacks and keep them in strategic spots at home and at work in case of hanger. Having trouble with vegetables? Throw them into a blender with berries or an apple and drink them.

Caffeine

Coffee and tea fans, rejoice. Repeated studies show that a small amount of caffeine is fine during pregnancy. In fact, *not* quitting cold turkey is better. The rebound headaches caused by stopping suddenly often require medication, and those medications can be worse than just sticking with your morning cup of joe. Caffeine, along with a tall glass of water, can help with headaches since you can't take ibuprofen or common NSAIDs.

There are downsides. Caffeine increases your blood pressure and heart rate (hey, the stimulation is the point, right?) and can cause you to feel more dehydrated. It also crosses the placenta, so your baby will feel some effect, though it doesn't cause a decrease in uterine blood flow or oxygenation. And caffeine is a diuretic, so more runs to the bathroom are in your future. In very large quantities, it is linked to miscarriage, low birth weights, and infertility.

So, what is the right amount? No more than two hundred milligrams of caffeine per day, which is about one twelve-ounce cup of brewed coffee or two espresso shots from your favorite barista. But here come the caveats: Each brew and drink type can have differing amounts. Also, soft drinks and energy drinks, chocolate and food items that contain coffee flavoring, and some OTC medications for pain relief, colds, and headaches have caffeine in them too, so factor those into your calculations.

WHAT NOT TO EAT

Okay, fine. If there is no universally right pregnancy diet, what about the things you *shouldn't* eat? Hearing that deli meat and sushi are off-limits, like so many things during this experience, triggers the inevitable question *Uh, why?* The answer: When not prepared or stored properly, they can carry harmful bacteria that cause complications and problems in your GI tract like food poisoning. Here are the most common culprits:

- Deli meat
- Undercooked, raw, and cured meats
- Soft or unpasteurized cheeses like Brie, Camembert, and blues (unpasteurized cheeses are rare in mainstream US grocery stores, but they do pop up at farmers' markets, so just check the labels)

- Pâtés and spreadable meats
- Raw eggs
- Unwashed raw produce
- High-mercury seafood (ahi tuna, shark, mackerel, tilefish, marlin)
- Unpasteurized juice or cider

Let's tackle deli meat first, since it's an odd one. Although things like roasted turkey, hot dogs, and chicken breasts are fully cooked before they're packaged or sliced, they are susceptible to a bacteria called listeria. Pregnant women's immune systems are suppressed while growing a human. While it will likely cause only a mild infection for you, listeriosis can cause serious issues for your baby, including miscarriage and stillbirth. Heating food to over 165 degrees Fahrenheit kills listeria, so if you're unable to resist that turkey sandwich, pop it in the oven or microwave before eating. Sadly, listeria can be found in veggies as well, so subscribe to an electronic alert on the CDC's website if you want outbreak updates.

Remember toxoplasmosis? It's not just caused by bacteria found in cat feces. You are more likely to contract it by eating raw and undercooked meats, which include fish, shellfish, and poultry. Toxoplasmosis can cause mental disabilities and blindness for your baby, so exercise caution and choose high-quality options if you are a lover of rare steaks or sushi.

E. coli and salmonella are the reasons you should skip the raw cookie dough, traditional Caesar dressing, and hollandaise. E. coli causes diarrhea, which can result in dehydration for you. But it is rarely linked to serious issues for the baby. Salmonella is similarly more a nuisance than harmful to your baby, but you should still take steps to avoid it. You can also contract salmonella through the skin of poultry and reptiles, so skip the petting zoo while pregnant, too.

So, let's recap:

- Keep your portion sizes reasonable (you aren't eating for two adult humans).
- Avoid processed foods and especially trans fats and added sugars whenever possible.
- Skip common food-poisoning culprits.
- Eat smaller, more frequent meals.
- Shoot for a mix of dairy, fat, and carbs from whole foods.
- Carry healthy snacks at all times (hunger and low blood sugar strike when you least expect it).
- **Do as best you can and don't beat yourself up over the occasional indulgence.**

Seriously, if you want a more specific dietary regimen, have at it with one of the thousands created by celebrities, mom bloggers, and nutritionists who have all discovered what they claim to be THE ONE. Following any of these to the letter is not possible unless you put in a lot of work cooking, avoid going out to eat, and never find yourself in a desperate moment of pregnancy hanger. Moderation is a more sustainable strategy.

Cooking is a favorite hobby of mine. But during pregnancy? Nope! A mere hint of red meat or fish smell sent me running to a different room. Aversions were more common than my cravings, and the unending acid reflux made it hard to eat much in one sitting, or late in the day.

In the first trimester, I avoided everything on the don't-eat list. But after that, if I was out for a nice meal, I occasionally indulged in a medium-rare steak or lamb and even had sushi. And though I generally ate well, there was a solid two-week phase of ice cream every night, and post–forty weeks, I devoured chocolate-chip cookies like it was my job.

EXERCISE

Exercise may be the last thing you want to think about while exhausted and nauseous. And it's even harder to get motivated later when you feel huge. Maybe you're also thinking, *Why bother? I'll just get back to it after the baby comes.*

Staying active during pregnancy is important. Any exercise, even walking, can boost your mood, keeps your weight in a healthy range, and can speed up recovery after birth. Labor and delivery are highly physical, and a strong body can make that process easier—and even shorter, in some cases. Not to mention that in the months leading up to birth, a little extra strength is helpful in carting around your growing bump.

It's not just about *your* health. Babies born to women who exercised a minimum of twenty minutes three times per week show more localized brain activity patterns in response to sounds, indicating their brains were becoming more efficient than those born to sedentary mothers. Exercising while pregnant may alter the vascular smooth tissue of infants and improve overall vascular function when they are adults, too.

With that in mind, we'll cover exercising safely with universally beneficial movements, treatments, and knowledge that will help your body stay healthy and help with aches and pains. All the exercises can be done at home with equipment that costs under $20, in whatever time you can devote to it.

If you were active before pregnancy, you can keep doing what you were doing before, with a few caveats: no high-impact activities that may result in a fall or jabs to the abdomen. These include skiing and snowboarding, horseback riding, scuba diving, skating, hockey, and basketball. Your blood volume will increase by 50 percent during pregnancy, which requires a lot more oxygen to maintain, so take your performance expectations down a notch. As things progress, you'll also need to make modifications to your movements, as your body just won't and can't contort itself into the same shapes anymore.

Not active before pregnancy? This isn't a call to join a gym, or the time to start training for a marathon. But unless your practitioner advises against it, try taking a few minutes (ideally a minimum of thirty) every day to walk as a start.

Tips for exercising safely

- **Abide by the talk test.** Heart rates aren't a reliable way to track whether you're going too hard, but breath is. If you can make understandable words while you exercise, you've passed the talk test.

- **Hydrate.** Water is your BFF during pregnancy, so drink a lot of it, more than you think you need.

- **Don't get overheated.** Sweating is fine, but in your first trimester especially, the surge of progesterone relaxes blood vessel walls, which lowers your blood pressure and increases your odds of light-headedness. So apologies, hot yoga enthusiasts—pregnancy is not the time for heated rooms.

- **Stretch.** Take a few minutes to warm up and cool down to avoid injury and maintain flexibility. Bonus points if you invest in a foam roller, which is basically like having access to an on-demand back rub. (More on foam rolling momentarily.)

- **When it's time to stop.** If you experience any bleeding, cramping, or reduced fetal movement while exercising, it's time to stop whatever you are doing and call your doctor.

One other thing to watch: that pesky little hormone relaxin. Its job is to relax your joints, tendons, ligaments, and muscle fibers and expand your rib cage and hips in preparation for birth. Relaxin levels peak during the first trimester and right before birth, so if you're in your favorite yoga class and can contort even more than usual, that's why. Because relaxin promotes more flexibility, be careful and don't overstretch.

Strength-training moves

Crunches and abdominal exercises that require going from lying down straight into a seated position are off-limits while pregnant. And after the first trimester, anything that requires lying flat on your back is neither comfortable nor recommended. But you can strengthen your obliques, butt, thighs, and other core muscle groups to help with labor and recovery, all from the comfort of home.

Before you start: If you do not feel comfortable doing this without supervision, or if any of these moves hurt, stop. If you aren't currently active, talk to your doctor before jumping into a new routine.

Cat/cow

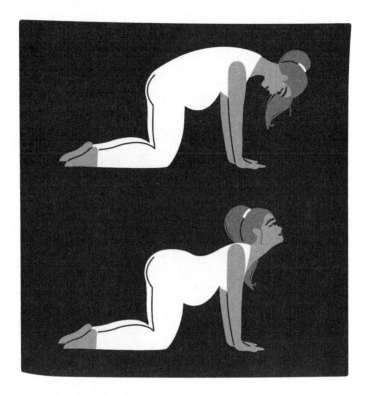

If you do yoga, this will be familiar.

- Get on your hands and knees.
- Your shoulders should be directly above your palms and your knees directly below your hips.
- Slowly lower your head and butt and round your spine toward the ceiling.
- Return to a neutral spine position.
- Arch your back and reach the top of your head and your tailbone upward.
- Return to a neutral spine position.
- Repeat ten times.

Squats

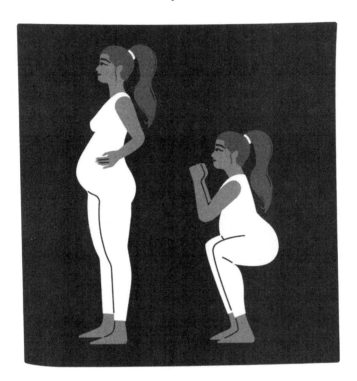

*You can do air squats or hold weights
in each hand to make it harder.*

- Stand with your feet hip-width apart with your toes facing forward and knees stacked above your toes.
- Bend your knees and reach back with your butt like you are sitting in a chair, keeping your chest and shoulders straight and upright.
- Stand back up.
- Repeat fifteen to twenty times.

Side planks

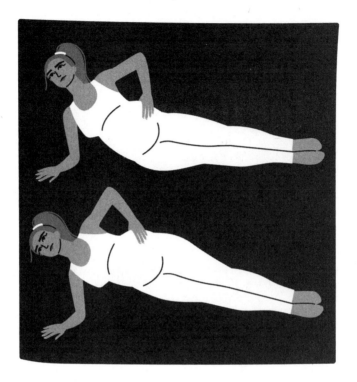

*Just because you can't crunch
doesn't mean you have to ignore your abs.*

- Lie on your side in a straight line.
- Make sure your elbow is directly under your shoulder, and your upper-body weight is resting on your forearm.
- Engaging your obliques, gently lift your hips off the floor, and hold, maintaining a neutral spine.
- For bonus points, lift and hold your top leg a few inches while your hips are raised.
- Do two or three rounds of thirty-to-sixty-second holds on each side.

Glute bridge

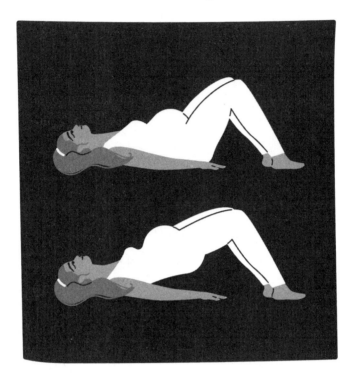

*A great one for anyone who sits
in front of a computer frequently.*

- Lie on your back with your knees bent and your knees and feet hip-width apart.
- Engage your core, squeeze your butt, and slowly lift your hips into a bridge.
- Hold, then slowly return your hips to the floor one vertebra at a time.
- Repeat eight to ten times.

Glute kickbacks

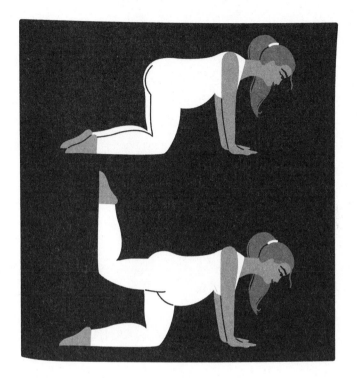

There are varying degrees of difficulty available;
make it your own.

- Get on your hands and knees.
- Your shoulders should be directly above your palms and your knees directly below your hips.
- Extend one leg out behind you and bend your knee at a 45-degree angle, keeping your abs engaged and your spine neutral and parallel with the floor.
- Hold for three to five seconds.
- Put your leg back on the floor and repeat with the other leg.
- For bonus points, raise the opposite arm straight out in front of you when you raise your leg.

Exercise was my sanity during those long months of on-and-off and finally on-again pregnancy. By stretching and staying active, I remained relatively free of pain and issues, and my recovery postpartum went quickly, even after a complicated birth.

So what did I do? The same things I did before I was pregnant. I started with strength training in the first two trimesters, modifying as needed. In the third, I added Pilates to help with my pelvic floor. Many times, I really didn't feel like working out and certainly couldn't maintain my previous pace. But I set a schedule, showed up, did as best I could, and always left feeling better than when I arrived. And boy, did my bump get some side-eye in those final months.

MANAGING ACHES AND PAINS

Maintaining a basic level of physical activity like walking helps with some of the inevitable body issues that arise during pregnancy. But as your center of gravity shifts and hormone levels jump up and down, a new crop of problems like sciatica (numbness or tingling in the legs), lower back pain, and even carpal tunnel can emerge. Rest is a prescription for some of this, but there are other ways to deal, such as getting outside help. Here are a few top tactics, including one you can do from home.

Bodywork and massage

Massage is the most common complementary therapy recommended during pregnancy, and for good reason. Massage decreases depression, anxiety, and pain, and can even lead to fewer prenatal complications. Women who experience depression during pregnancy may benefit the most from massage, as the rates of prematurity and low birth weight drop along with their cortisol levels.

Outside of helping you feel pampered during pregnancy, massage has big benefits during labor. Women who received massage therapy reported labors that were three hours shorter on average, and less need for medication.

Before you run out and book a massage, there are a few things to know. Many therapists will not do it in the first trimester due to a fear of stimulating labor-inducing acupressure points, a worry that is not actually grounded in science. That said, if you're on the conservative side or have a complicated pregnancy, you may want to wait for the full-body rubdown until you are farther along into the second trimester.

When booking a massage, no matter how early you are, let your therapist know you are pregnant. They won't tell your whole social circle, and it's important for them to be able to customize your treatment based on how many weeks into pregnancy you are. This includes preparing the all-important pregnancy cushion that has a hole in the middle specifically to cradle your bump. Side-lying is another option if you're not into the way that feels.

Foam rolling

Bodywork and massage are amazing, but doing it daily or even weekly is tough. To the uninitiated, the thought of using a piece of foam to loosen up probably sounds strange. And in the third trimester, it isn't easy. There are tools like the tiger tail or self-massage stick for the final stretch if you catch the bug. But until then, foam rolling is an excellent way to give yourself a less invasive type of home massage and release the tension in your growing body, all for as little as $5.

If you sit in front of a computer or are in the car all day or, I don't know, are carting around an extra human for nine months, your muscles develop knots and adhesions. Fascia, the thin band of tissue that holds your organs, bones, nerve fibers, and muscles in place can get tight during pregnancy and cause pain too. Foam rolling provides myofascial release, which relaxes these contracted muscles and tissue. It can also improve blood and lymphatic circulation and even your sleep.

Foam rollers come in a variety of densities and sizes. Beginners generally like a softer, less dense roll. The truly hard core go with versions that feature spikes. A foam roller's greatest feature may be convenience. No going to a gym or spa, or waiting for your partner to offer up their services. Keep it by your bed, TV, or anywhere that provides a visual reminder and a little space. At first, myofascial release can be uncomfortable, especially if you are releasing a particularly tight area. Be careful and gentle and stop any movement if you are not able to balance on the roller. YouTube has many videos that show exactly how it works if you need in-depth guidance.

To get the most out of your rolling session, hydrate, go slow, and breathe through your movements. There are a few areas of your aching pregnant body that can really benefit from foam rolling: your outer thighs, or IT bands; your calves; and your lower back.

The basics of foam rolling:

- Sit on the floor or a yoga mat with your foam roller.
- Target a specific sore muscle and position the roller directly underneath it.
- Find a comfortable, stable position with a neutral spine.
- Use your body weight to roll over that area slowly five to ten times. When it feels good, pause and give it a moment to really sink in.

I still keep a foam roller by my bed. I used it before and after exercise and long walks, and every night before I went to sleep while pregnant. In fact, I enjoyed myofascial release so much that I went to see a massage therapist who specialized in it. She debugged a pinched nerve, unstuck my pelvis on more than one occasion, and generally helped me stay comfortable. She also won the award for best business name: Muscle Butter.

Acupuncture

Acupuncture is a branch of Chinese medicine that uses thin needles to stimulate specific points on the body. Depending on where the needles are placed, you might feel relaxed or energized, or experience localized effects in one area. It may inspire the body to produce endorphins, the hormones that provide natural pain relief. It's also possible that it stimulates the nervous system or changes how pain is perceived. We don't know exactly why or how acupuncture works, which leads people to sometimes question its efficacy or put it squarely in the woo category. Another reason is that acupuncture follows a different understanding of the human body versus Western medicine, and as a result, few studies are published in traditional medical journals.

Due to its effects on the hypothalamus-pituitary-ovarian (HPO) axis, acupuncture is often used to improve hormone-related problems. The HPO axis is responsible for production of FSH (follicle-stimulating hormone), which stimulates ovarian follicles to grow and mature, and LH (luteinizing hormone), which stimulates ovulation. During pregnancy, it can diminish many of the annoying aches and symptoms, and later reduce pain during labor.

If you want to give it a whirl, look for clinics that specialize in fertility or women's health. Appointments begin with a general health update, a check-in on existing or new symptoms, and specific goals for your treatment. Acupuncturists receive training across many modalities of Chinese medicine, so they'll also suggest lifestyle and nutrition modifications. After the needle insertion, you'll be left for fifteen to forty-five minutes so the treatment can do its magic. It's a great time for a quick but epic nap, as the points acupuncture targets help you to relax. That alone is a reason for you to try it if you're feeling anxious and nothing else is working.

Many practices accept insurance, which means you'll either have a copay or be reimbursed for the full treatment cost later. Like doulas, it can be a pregnancy benefit via your employer too.

I was skeptical the first time I tried acupuncture to help manage pain related to a sports injury. Especially as I am not great (okay, fine—I'm terrible) with needles. But it didn't hurt and was more effective pain relief than anything my doctor prescribed. While it's unclear whether acupuncture had a direct impact on my fertility, an indisputable benefit during pregnancy was helping me through the rough patches. Having a weekly check-in with my acupuncturist followed by a relaxing break eased a lot of my anxiety and provided the emotional support I didn't even know I needed— a therapy session followed by a short, restorative nap.

TO TEST
OR NOT TO TEST?

Making sense of prenatal testing

Your baby may not be ready for the SAT, but their first tests happen before they exit the womb. And they aren't the only one under the microscope. You'll be treated to what feels like a never-ending battery of pricks, pokes, prods, and blood draws during pregnancy, too.

It's easy to jump down a rabbit hole of things that could possibly go wrong, so here's a reminder that most babies are born without any problems. Unless medically indicated, many of the testing options below are just that—options. You have full control over which tests are performed, and what information you receive. That said, unless you really hate needles (or peeing), there isn't much downside to your tests, as most are noninvasive. Most practitioners will insist you keep up with blood panels each trimester and gestational diabetes and group B strep (GBS) screenings at a minimum.

The bigger decision is how much information you want about your growing baby. Prenatal testing looks for abnormalities that indicate developmental or physical problems. It starts with screenings that calculate the likelihood that the baby might have a condition and progresses as needed to diagnostic tests that provide a definitive answer. If you have no family history, are low risk, and everything looks fine, you probably won't be offered prenatal testing, though you can still opt in. If testing isn't called for and you still want to do it, insurance seldom covers it.

Some couples choose to forgo testing entirely. Others want to know every detail. Most will at least do ultrasounds, if only to get their first peeks at the baby and to learn its gender. But prenatal testing isn't perfect and can cause a lot of stress. There can be false negatives and positives, and diagnostic testing carries risks.

If you're weighing what's right for you, ask what you would do with the information you receive. Good news gives peace of mind. Bad news is more complicated. Knowing in advance that your baby will require special help or surgery gives you time to plan, and in some cases the opportunity to manage conditions before birth. But you may be faced with decisions you never expect to make, like dealing with a result that reveals a severe or even fatal condition. If you know you would do nothing differently regardless of the results, testing may not be for you.

PRENATAL TESTING FOR BABY

Ultrasounds

For many parents, the first ultrasound is when pregnancy starts to feel real, especially after showing friends and family your keepsake sonogram. But wait, isn't a sonogram the same thing as an ultrasound? Though the words are sometimes used interchangeably, an ultrasound is the procedure itself, and the resulting photo is the sonogram.

Inspired by echolocation in bats and the sound waves used to search for the *Titanic*, ultrasound first entered prenatal care in 1956. Dr. Ian Donald of Glasgow was the first to use it in obstetric practice, but it didn't catch on in the US for another twenty years. It's now a standard of prenatal care around the world.

Ultrasound uses high-frequency sound waves to make images of the inside of the body. During pregnancy, the probe directs these sound waves through the cold gel on your stomach into your uterus. When the waves make contact with the fetus, they bounce back and create a picture. Ultrasound is used to make sure a baby is growing properly, to estimate gestational age, to check organ development and blood flow, and, of course, to discover the gender. Only two ultrasounds happen during a routine pregnancy—one in the first trimester and another in the second, known as the anatomy scan. If you are carrying multiples, have bleeding, or are considered high risk, more will be scheduled.

Before you get sad about the dearth of ultrasounds, remember that it is a diagnostic procedure, not a baby peep show. Skip the at-home Doppler to listen to your baby's heartbeat unless your ob-gyn or midwife asks you to. It can be easy to miss fetal movement and hard to find the heartbeat. Same goes for predicting whose nose she has with 3-D and 4-D ultrasounds. The risks of too much ultrasound exposure haven't been studied, so minimizing the number you receive is best.

So what exactly are the risks of ultrasounds? At very high power, ultrasound waves can damage human tissue. We aren't sure exactly how high, because it isn't ethical to subject anyone to that testing. What about radiation? X-rays and other medical imaging use ionizing radiation, which removes electrons from atoms and molecules. The nonionizing radiation used in ultrasound technology does not. When administered infrequently and performed in a medical context by a trained professional, ultrasounds are considered safe.

Your first ultrasound usually happens between eight and ten weeks. It confirms the fetal heartbeat, checks dating, ensures the pregnancy is happening in the uterus (as opposed to the fallopian tubes, which is the dangerous condition with a misleading name covered earlier, ectopic pregnancy), and reveals if you are (surprise!) growing more than one human. This is the only time in your pregnancy that your due date can shift slightly, as measurements of fetal age are more reliable in the first trimester than at any other time.

A second ultrasound can take place between eleven and fourteen weeks, as part of the first-trimester combined screening. Also known as the nuchal translucency screening, it combines measurements of the fluid at the base of the fetus's neck with results from a blood test to estimate the likelihood of genetic conditions like Down syndrome. The fluid in the nuchal fold is visible only during this period, while the tissue is still translucent.

The anatomy scan in the second trimester happens between eighteen and twenty weeks and is your first real peek at your baby. During the thirty-to-forty-five-minute session, your baby's head and trunk will be measured, and the weight will be estimated. The scan also checks amniotic fluid levels and the state and location of the placenta, and the baby's kidneys, bladder, stomach, brain, spine, and sex organs. If you don't want to know the gender, tell your sonographer before they start. It's easy to see the presence (or absence) of a penis at this point.

Ultrasounds are only used later in pregnancy to monitor higher-risk women, so if yours is progressing without any issues, expect the anatomy scan to be your last. If you were hoping to get a preview of your baby's size and weight, measurements taken in the third trimester are not very accurate and can be off by as many as one or two pounds.

Noninvasive prenatal screening (NIPS)

Your baby's presence isn't confined to your uterus. Just as an explosion of toys in your house will later register your child's existence, their residency in your body is evident everywhere, by way of your bloodstream. Fetal placental fragments are detectable in your blood as early as ten weeks and are the basis for NIPS, also sometimes called cell-free DNA screening tests or cfDNA tests. These fetal placental fragments, which match the baby's DNA, are sampled and analyzed to screen for genetic conditions and chromosomal abnormalities, primarily trisomies, or the presence of extra chromosomes and sex chromosome aneuploidies. Because the test screens sex chromosomes, it can also reveal the sex of your baby.

The result you'll receive from NIPS is the likelihood that a fetus might have a particular condition, not a definitive diagnosis. NIPS requires a diagnostic test like CVS or amniocentesis to confirm the result. Although it was first recommended for high-risk patients, NIPS is now offered to nearly everyone, as it produces fewer false positives than the quad screen and because it's noninvasive.

NIPS are not regulated by the FDA, which means that it is very important to work with your provider and only use tests that they trust. Some NIPS marketed as "premium" or "advanced" claim to screen for even more rare genetic conditions but are not always accurate and can give an alarming percentage of false positives.

How is it done?
Blood draw

When is it done?
Ten weeks or later, with results in seven to fourteen days

What does it test?
Most versions screen only for three main chromosomal conditions—trisomy 13, trisomy 18, and trisomy 21 (Down syndrome)—and sex chromosome abnormalities, which is how it reveals the baby's gender. Other genetic markers are still being evaluated for accuracy, so you probably will not see them in your results.

Who should get it?
Anyone can get this test, and it is increasingly offered regardless of your risk factors. It is recommended for women who have a high-risk pregnancy, are over thirty-five, or have had a previous pregnancy with a chromosomal abnormality.

Advantages
It's a noninvasive blood test, so there is no risk of miscarriage or complication. If the results come back normal, you likely will not

need to move on to diagnostic testing. You can also elect to find out the gender months before the twenty-week anatomy scan.

Disadvantages

Screening tests are not diagnostic, meaning they cannot tell you with 100 percent certainty if your baby is going to be affected by any of these conditions. It assigns odds based on the presence or absence of extra chromosomal matter. If the screening is positive, your doctor will suggest a CVS or amnio to confirm. There can be false positives, especially in low-risk pregnancies. If you are looking for the most data possible, CVS and amnio can diagnose hundreds of conditions; NIPS screens for only four.

Second-trimester quadruple screening (quad screen)

The quad screen provides your baby's risk profile for certain genetic disorders and birth defects like Down syndrome and spina bifida (failure of the neural tube along the spine to close fully). If you've already cleared a first-trimester screening, it may not be offered. But in some pregnancies, findings from multiple screenings are combined to improve the detection rate of some conditions.

How is it done?

Blood draw

When is it done?

Fifteen to twenty-two weeks

What does it test?

Four different markers in the pregnant woman's blood: alpha-fetoprotein (AFP), estriol, inhibin A, and hCG

Who should get it?

Women with positive first-trimester screening, or NIPS results, or anyone who started prenatal care later in pregnancy

Advantages

The quad screen is noninvasive, and a negative result decreases the likelihood you will need diagnostic tests like amnio or CVS.

Disadvantages

The quad screen does have false positives and negatives and, like all screenings, gives you the chance of a condition, not a guarantee. If you have a positive screen, you'll speak to a genetic counselor who will advise which diagnostic test is appropriate to provide a definite answer.

Chorionic villus sampling (CVS)

Chorionic villi are tiny hairlike projections found in the placenta that route nutrients, oxygen, and antibodies from you to your baby. They also hold fetal cells that contain your baby's chromosomes and DNA.

The procedure removes these fetal cells from the placenta, where it attaches to the uterine wall. CVS is a conclusive diagnostic test and can be done as early as ten weeks. It can confirm positive NIPS or NT screening results and check for inherited disorders and serves as an earlier alternative to amniocentesis.

How is it done?

CVS can be performed two ways—transabdominally, with a needle inserted through the abdomen, or transcervically, via a small tube inserted through the cervix. Using ultrasound guidance, a sample of chorionic villi are suctioned or drawn from the placenta.

The procedure can be uncomfortable, and some women experience cramping for several days afterward.

When is it done?

It's the earliest available diagnostic test, done between ten and thirteen weeks. Results can come back in a few days, or weeks, depending on how many tests are run.

What does it test?

Hundreds of different genetic and chromosomal conditions. It also reveals the gender.

Who should get it?

CVS is offered only if there is an increased risk of genetic or chromosomal conditions, mostly due to a positive NIPS screening or a family or medical history.

Advantages

CVS is done earlier in pregnancy than amniocentesis and results come back quickly.

Disadvantages

CVS carries a less than 1 percent chance of miscarriage, and transcervical CVS can cause vaginal bleeding. Rates of miscarriage between transcervical and transabdominal procedures are the same. Sometimes the sample cells are not suitable for testing, so the procedure may need to be repeated. Unlike amniocentesis, CVS cannot detect neural tube or anatomical defects.

Amniocentesis

German doctors first pioneered the technique behind amniocentesis in the 1880s to relieve excess amniotic pressure on a growing fetus.

The amnio hit the medical mainstream in the 1950s and is the most well-known of the prenatal diagnostic tests. It can diagnose everything from genetic abnormalities and fetal lung maturity to infection through a sample of amniotic fluid. Amniotic fluid's main job is to cushion and protect the baby in the womb, and to help regulate temperature. But it also contains fetal cells and proteins, which is what an amniocentesis analyzes. It was used more frequently when there were fewer testing options, and due to the risks involved, should be used only if indicated.

How is it done?

Using ultrasound guidance, your doctor will insert a thin needle into the amniotic sac away from the baby. A small sample of amniotic fluid is withdrawn, then sent to a lab and examined for genetic abnormalities. There can be stinging and cramping during the procedure, and it can cause discomfort afterward, so you'll want to relax for the rest of the day.

When is it done?

Typically fifteen to twenty weeks into a pregnancy, with results back in two weeks.

What does it test?

Many different birth defects and genetic conditions, from cystic fibrosis and Tay-Sachs disease to neural tube defects like anencephaly, which CVS cannot detect.

Who should get it?

Women with abnormal ultrasounds, genetic screenings, or lab results, previous pregnancies or children with birth defects, a high-risk pregnancy, an infection like toxoplasmosis, or a family history of genetic or birth defects. It is also used to test for paternity.

Advantages

Amniocentesis is over 99 percent accurate in detecting genetic disorders and 90 percent accurate for neural tube defects.

Disadvantages

As with CVS, there is a less than 1 percent chance of miscarriage, and rare complications like preterm labor, leaking amniotic fluid, needle injury, and infection. Sometimes the test must be repeated if the sample cannot be accurately tested. And though it is highly accurate, amnio cannot detect every single possible condition, or the severity, so there is still a chance that even with a normal result your baby will be born with a defect the test didn't find.

TESTS JUST FOR YOU

These tests don't come until later in your pregnancy, but in the spirit of giving you an easy way to reference them later, we'll cover them all in one spot.

Rhesus (Rh) factor blood test

Named for the rhesus monkey, which also carries the gene, Rh factor is a type of protein found on the surface of red blood cells. If you have the protein, you are Rh positive. Don't have it? You are Rh negative. Eighty-five percent of people are Rh positive, and the only way your baby can be negative is for each parent to have at least one negative factor.

An incompatibility isn't a problem for you. But it is for your baby, as your immune system will perceive the baby to be a foreign object and attack. Left unaddressed, the incompatibility can cause hemolytic anemia, which causes your baby's red blood cells to be destroyed faster than they can be replaced. It can also lead to jaundice and to liver and heart failure.

This screen is usually part of the blood draw at your first prenatal visit, so the incompatibility is easy to detect and treat. If you are found to be Rh negative, you'll be given Rh immunoglobulin at twenty-eight weeks, and within seventy-two hours of birth.

Glucose screening

The second-trimester glucose screening happens between twenty-four and twenty-eight weeks and is performed to see if you have developed gestational diabetes mellitus (GDM). It may be done in the first trimester if you have a history of diabetes or other risk factors. The standard format: a blood test before and after you chug a small container of very sugary water. Your blood glucose will be measured before and an hour after the sugar bomb hits, and if the level is high, you'll move on to a three-hour glucose tolerance test. The three-hour version is similar but requires an overnight fast. Your blood sugar is measured before you drink the same drink, and then again once an hour for three hours. If your readings are still high, you will be diagnosed with gestational diabetes.

Between 2 and 10 percent of pregnancies are affected by GDM, and if yours is one of them, it's not your fault. It's also not due to the excess carbs you ate enduring first-trimester morning sickness, or the croissant you wolfed down the day before your test. Being of certain races and ethnicities, genetics, and a family history can all increase the risk of developing GDM. Most women can manage their blood sugar levels through monitoring, diet, and exercise, and are often referred to a Registered Dietitian Nutritionist who specializes in diabetes for extra support during and after pregnancy. In some cases, insulin or metformin, both of which are pregnancy-safe, will be prescribed, as are continuous glucose monitors. Keeping gestational diabetes under control is important, since the condition increases your odds of having a larger-than-average baby, C-section, stillbirth, or preterm birth.

Gestational diabetes goes away after birth, but 50 percent of those affected develop type 2 diabetes later. For that reason, your levels will be checked postdelivery, then monitored every three years.

I was never happy about the sugar-high crash aspect of this test. Glucola, the sugary beverage used for this test, is objectively gross, and there should be a better option (please someone work on this!). But this test is recommended by every major medical organization, and gestational diabetes is important to detect and monitor— please don't skip it.

Group B strep (GBS)

Yes, we're jumping ahead a bit with this one. Done during the third trimester, between thirty-six and thirty-eight weeks, the group B strep test is a simple swab test of the vagina and perineum. GBS is a normal bacterium in the vagina (about one in four women carry it), but it can be passed to your baby on its way out during birth. If that happens, it can cause severe lung, brain, and blood infections. Left untreated, there's a one in two hundred chance of infection, and a 5 percent chance of infant death. If you are GBS positive and have a vaginal delivery, you'll be given IV antibiotics. C-section moms do not need antibiotics unless the amniotic sac has ruptured.

During the second pregnancy, we did an NIPS at ten weeks, both because it's standard for those of us over thirty-five, and to reduce the need for invasive diagnostic tests. When the genetic counselor called to say the NIPS was positive for trisomy 18, we had no idea what it was. It was not news we wanted. Also known as Edwards syndrome, trisomy 18 is a fatal developmental condition that most often ends in stillbirth.

We were devastated.

NIPS is not a diagnostic test, so we had to confirm the result with a CVS. Walking into a waiting room full of happy pregnant bumps and new babies made test day even more difficult. The CVS itself was also very unpleasant (it felt like being pinched from the inside), but the silent, joyless ultrasound was worse. I sobbed from the time I entered the room until we left.

The CVS results and dire ultrasound findings showed that our best-case scenario was miscarriage within weeks. Not wanting to believe we were out of options, I called a genetics expert friend to vet the efficacy of the tests, and a neonatologist to fully understand our options. They all confirmed that there was no possibility of a happy ending. It was over.

Terminating a very wanted pregnancy, even under those circumstances, was the hardest experience of my life.

The day of the procedure, it took a full morning for my cervix to ripen; the actual dilation and curettage (D&C) took only thirty minutes. The dilation was uncomfortable, but other than feeling groggy and emotionally drained, there was very little pain after. The next day, every pregnancy symptom was gone. And after twenty-four hours of light spotting, it felt like the whole thing never happened.

After our two-month hiatus, I was pregnant. Again. The first cycle we tried. Nick and I agreed not to obsess about what could go wrong and let it be. We knew we were lucky to get pregnant so easily; now we just had to wait.

This time, we cleared the NIPS and, since everything was normal, did not opt into diagnostic testing. While I had (many) moments of anxiety, we decided to follow the process and not seek out more information than we needed. The first trimester was tough emotionally, but physically, this pregnancy was much easier from the start. Maybe because I had more perspective. Perhaps because I was full of so much love for the people who surrounded us while we struggled. Certainly because I had no morning sickness. And definitely because I stopped white-knuckling and trying to control the process.

I know this wasn't easy to read—believe me, it was excruciating to write and relive. But this experience inspired the book you now hold in your hands. I hope that by sharing my story, I can help anyone in a similar situation to feel less alone than I did.

First-Trimester Checklist

- [ ] Create a budget for pregnancy and the first year.
- [ ] Check your personal products for ingredients that are not pregnancy-safe.
- [ ] Go over your supplements and medications with your practitioner (if you didn't during conception).
- [ ] Look into complementary practices to support your pregnancy emotionally and physically.
- [ ] Try to relax; eat moderately and focus on whole, unprocessed foods; hydrate; exercise as your body allows—even if it's just a quick walk.
- [ ] Start discussions about if, when, and how to return to work, college savings, will(s) and trust(s), and advanced healthcare directives.
- [ ] Talk about prenatal testing with your partner.

The Second Trimester

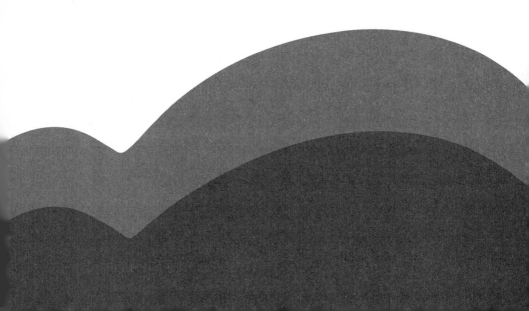

You can breathe a small sigh of relief when you make it into the second trimester, first because your risk of miscarriage drops, and because you will start feeling more like yourself (though you may not look it for long). Enjoy those deep breaths while you can, as you'll be huffing and puffing as that growing baby starts to crowd your lungs. In the good-news column, the spending-half-your-pregnancy-looking-and-feeling-chubby-and-bloated-but-not-actually-pregnant phase—especially if it's your first—finally comes to an end.

The second trimester is the crowd favorite, as the legion pregnancy symptoms taper off, and your bump is a cute but manageable size. It's a great time to take a babymoon and plow through tasks like putting together the nursery. You can also learn your baby's gender if you haven't already, and will feel the first flutters of movement, which make the whole thing feel less theoretical.

Around twenty-two weeks I no longer looked like I'd just eaten a burrito (but all the time) and had an actual bump. Though I was still a little (okay, a lot) absentminded, my energy returned, and I could make it through a whole day (and to as late as 9:00 p.m., a huge accomplishment) without a nap.

Full disclosure: After spending two-thirds of a year stuck in the first trimester, I was not a fan of pregnancy. The exhaustion, the super-smell, the night peeing—I was sick of the whole thing. But then . . . the kicking started and the experience became much less abstract. There was a real, live human zooming around my abdomen like a little mango-size goldfish. A male goldfish, as it turned out. Once I stopped replaying that scene from Alien *every time I felt a flutter, it was pretty cool.*

SO WHAT'S HAPPENING IN THERE?

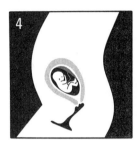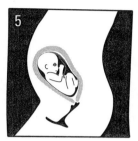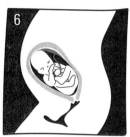

Month 4

Baby: This month is all about moving and grooving and beginning to put on some fat. At five to six inches long, the baby is around the size of a clenched fist and is practicing breathing, sucking, and swallowing. They will start to look less like a creature from outer space and more like a human, as the ears move from the neck to the sides of the head, and their eyes get closer together. Though their body is still skinny, the baby fat you won't be able to stop pinching later begins to form along with the lungs.

You: Thus conclude many of the first-trimester symptoms you've grown to love. Your morning sickness should dwindle, the night peeing will diminish, and generally you should start to feel better. Your sex drive may also return, accompanied by new symptoms like heartburn and breathlessness. The first fetal movements, also called the quickening, are detectable this month too. They can be more like flutters or indigestion, so don't feel left out if it takes a while to discern the difference. Your swelling abdomen will finally start to look more bump-like, which means pants sans elastic will be less and less appealing by the day.

Month 5

Baby: This is the magic month when, if you don't know already and want to, the gender can be revealed on ultrasound. Reproductive organs are forming along with a unique set of fingerprints, and your baby is just beginning to perceive the difference between light and dark—though their eyes are still fused shut. A cheese-like substance called vernix caseosa now coats their skin to protect it from pruning in the amniotic fluid. Your baby nearly doubles in size this month, starting at five inches and five ounces and growing to ten inches and nearly a pound by the start of month six.

You: Rejoice, you're halfway done with pregnancy! Your belly is starting to pop, and so may your belly button this month. How much you show depends entirely on your pregnancy and build—there is no standard size—so try not to compare if you're bumpin' more or less than what you see in your feeds. Pregnancy brain may cause you to forget things here and there (this symptom sticks around long after birth, sadly). The extra size and weight of the baby mean your breathlessness will increase as your lungs get pushed up, and your appetite may expand to keep up with the baby's growing demands. So may bloating and other delightful digestive issues.

Month 6

Baby: It's time to pack on the pounds. Your baby will go from roughly one pound to two by the end of this month and be about the size of a bowling pin. This month is all about growth— growing fat deposits, organs, bones, muscle, and even eyebrows and vocal cords. Movements will become more pronounced and easier to detect this month, and you may experience the first of many run-ins with in utero hiccups. Hearing also picks up, which means loud noises can trigger their startle reflex.

You: Think of month six as the sequel to month five. You'll experience many of the same changes, mostly in the form of your abdomen stretching to a basketball-like size. Your swelling size can also mean more aches and pains and retaining fluid in your ankles and feet. Symptoms like bleeding gums, constipation, heartburn, and mysterious leg cramps can also intensify. Now is the time to watch your stress levels, as pregnancy-related hypertension can start, too.

I had one full-on fall-on-my-face fainting spell at a crowded party entering the second trimester, and other close calls in warm spaces. Dressing in layers is the best antidote to wildly vacillating pregnancy temperature swings.

Second-trimester symptoms and solutions

Skin Changes

- **When does it happen?**
  Typically at the beginning of the second trimester, can be earlier

- **Symptoms**
  Linea nigra (dark line down your abdomen), melasma (dark patches on your face), stretch marks

- **Cause**
  Hormonal changes cause increased melanin in the skin

- Solutions

They usually fade after delivery, but stay out of the sun whenever possible and use sunscreen to minimize the effects. Moisturizer can help the appearance of stretch marks and related itchiness but will not prevent them.

Insomnia

- When does it happen?

Four in five women experience insomnia at some point during pregnancy. It can start during the first trimester but usually intensifies over time.

- Symptoms

Inability to sleep through the night, waking up frequently

- Cause

Increasing bump size, night peeing, anxiety, vivid dreams, hormones, heartburn, and back pain

- Solutions

Invest in a body pillow, take a warm bath, or ask your partner for a massage. Pretend you're in the womb and test-drive white-noise or relaxation apps. Shorten your naps to thirty minutes or less so they don't interfere with your sleep schedule. Exercise.

Leg cramps and restless legs

- When does it happen?

Can strike at any time, but more common later into pregnancy, especially common at night

- Symptoms

  Calf cramps, restless feeling in legs, inability to get comfortable

- Cause

  Unclear, but thought to be related to fatigue, dehydration, or a calcium or magnesium deficiency

- Solutions

  Exercise and walk, bath or hot shower, massage, calf raises, compression stockings, and drinking water. Ask your practitioner about taking a magnesium supplement.

Stuffy nose

- When does it happen?

  Increases throughout pregnancy, but can start anytime

- Symptoms

  Runny or bloody nose, congestion

- Cause

  Swollen mucous membranes thanks to the increased blood levels in your body

- Solutions

  Saline rinses or drops (neti pot), humidifier, sleep with your head elevated

Dizziness

- When does it happen?
  Increases throughout pregnancy, but can start anytime

- Symptoms
  Light-headedness, dizziness, fainting

- Cause
  Changes in circulation

- Solutions
  Avoid standing for long periods of time, drink plenty of fluids, and stand up slowly.

Bleeding gums (a.k.a. pregnancy gingivitis)

- When does it happen?
  Typically starts in the second trimester and persists until birth

- Symptoms
  Sensitive or bleeding gums

- Cause
  Hormonal changes cause increased sensitivity to the bacteria in plaque

- Solutions
  Rinse with salt water, brush with a softer toothbrush, and keep flossing (even though it kind of sucks).

Round ligament pain

- **When does it happen?**

  As your bump expands and grows, different for everyone

- **Symptoms**

  Crampy or achy feelings in your lower abdomen while exercising, sneezing, laughing, or getting out of bed

- **Cause**

  Muscles and ligaments stretching to support the growing uterus

- **Solutions**

  Get up and down slowly, and try a belly-support band or belt. As always, listen to your body. If it happens while you exercise, or after any other specific movement, switch up the routine.

WHAT DO I ACTUALLY NEED TO BUY?

Building a minimalist baby registry and not going broke purchasing maternity clothes

If you haven't started a budget, now is a good time to start, as the expenses will grow along with your bump to go beyond prenatal care and weird food cravings. Your body is going through some major changes, and some of the prepregnancy clothes you've worn until now will stretch to the limit or go away until after the postpartum period. Have no fear—there are plenty of ways to hack maternity clothes and incorporate flattering pieces without buying a new wardrobe.

Maternity clothes aren't the only purchases to plan during the second trimester. You'll also want to start picking away at a nursery and compile a baby registry, especially if someone in your life wants to throw a party or shower you and your new addition with love. Read on for a full list of vetted items along with guidance from seasoned parents. The main one: Take it easy and don't buy too much before you get to know your baby.

A GUIDE TO BUYING BABY GEAR

In Finland, every mother leaves the hospital with a box of items her new addition absolutely needs in the first thirty days of life. This tradition goes back to 1938, when the box was created for low-income families to help with the terrible infant mortality rate—at that time, sixty-five out of every thousand babies died in their first year of life. To qualify, all pregnant women had to do was attend a prenatal appointment in the first trimester. The combined health and free-stuff initiative was so effective it was rolled out to the rest of the population in 1949 and continues today.

So what's in this box? Well, to start with, even the box is part of the package, as it can be the baby's first crib, provided to prevent newborn co-sleeping. The other items include a mattress and cover, sleeping bag, undersheet, duvet, blanket, clothes in various weights and sizes, diapers and wipes, nail scissors, hairbrush, toothbrush, thermometer, diaper cream, washcloth, hooded bath towel, book and teething toy, bra pads, and condoms.

Minimalist baby registry

Though there are a few things missing, the reality is, for the first thirty days anyway, *babies just don't need that much stuff.* Also, your baby may not like that must-have swing your friend's baby lived in, so when it comes to bigger items that are only useful for a few months, try to borrow what you can.

This configuration has been working for the mothers of Finland for the past eighty-plus years, so consider this list, to borrow a software term, your minimum viable registry. We're going with the word *registry* as even if you aren't having a baby shower, it's a handy way to track what you need and what you've already purchased. A few bonus items are thrown in because, let's face it, friends and family will want to buy you nonessential cute stuff, too.

- Infant-safe car seat
- Stroller (make sure your car seat is compatible)
- Safe place for baby to sleep (bassinet, pack 'n' play, or crib)
- Mattress, mattress cover, and a fitted sheet for crib
- Swaddling blankets
- Diaper bag (or organizer insert)
- Pacifiers (two types)
- Changing table or pad
- Diapers (average ten changes daily, so 320 will get you through the first month)
- Wipes
- Burp cloths (you can never have too many)
- Bibs
- Clothes (in a variety of sizes beyond newborn)
    - Onesies (wide head openings and loose legs)
    - One-piece pajamas
    - Socks
    - Hats
    - Dress-up outfits for going home, birth announcements, etc.
    - For a winter baby, two blanket sleepers, no-scratch mittens, a bunting bag, warm hat
- Rattle, teething ring, and a few other infant-safe toys
- Books
- Nursing pillow (especially if you have a C-section)
- Baby soap and shampoo
- Hooded baby towel/robe combo
- Grooming kit (brush, nail clippers and file, thermometer)
- First-aid kit
- Nasal aspirator
- Aquaphor (for diaper rash prevention and cuts)

If breastfeeding:

- Breast pads
- Nipple butter or lanolin
- Breast pump
- Pumping bra
- Breast milk storage containers

If formula feeding:

- Two different bottle types with age-appropriate nipples
- Newborn-friendly formula
- Bottle-washing soap and drying rack

Nonessential but great:

- Comfortable chair for feedings
- Diaper-disposal receptacle
- Floor gym/play mat (for tummy time)
- Baby monitor
- Night-light
- White-noise machine
- Infant carrier or wrap
- Baby bathtub

Purchasing pro tips

When it comes to brands and models, everyone's preferences and aesthetics are different. What follows is the collected wisdom of parents to help inform your purchasing decisions.

- Newborn clothes fit only for the first few weeks (if they fit at all—hello, ten-pound babies!). Sizes are not consistent across different brands either, so one company's 3 to 6 months may be another's 0 to 3. Request a variety of sizes on your registry, so your tiny human has fun clothes for the first year and beyond.

- Optimize for clothing that is easy to put on and take off. A few features to look for: items that snap at the bottom, zip, or have magnets.
- Share a photo of the nursery and color scheme or include (and mark "purchased") things you buy so family who inevitably goes off-list knows what you have.
- To get home from the hospital, you need an infant-safe car seat. Yes, the hospital may check to make sure you have one and that it's installed correctly before allowing you to leave the premises. And yes, there are professional car seat installers.
- Wipe warmers are popular, but ask yourself: Do you want to haul it around when you are on the go? Getting a baby used to toasty wipes means they will be more likely to scream in public when the mobile version is cold.
- The towels and washcloths you already own are fine for your baby, too. That said, hooded towels (especially those with animal ears) are adorable.
- Get to know your baby before buying a metric ton of diapers (or anything else in bulk). Their build and preferences mean some of the things you purchase just won't work or fit, and some brands leak.

Beyond individual items, the best high-level tip is to try to be the happy recipient of hand-me-down items and look in consignment shops for lightly worn baby clothes. Your baby will not know the difference. Larger items like cribs, pack 'n' plays, swings, and carriers are often up for grabs from those transitioning to the toddler years or finally clearing out storage spaces.

Seriously, don't buy it all in advance, and beware of different brands and their completely random sizing. We used newborn clothes for one week before my son outgrew them. A European brand I love must have used mice to size their clothes, as he was too big for twelve-month onesies at ten weeks.

To my dismay, my son didn't much care for being worn in a wrap or sling, so in those early weeks we depended on a bouncer and cushion that looked sort of like a pool float during his waking hours. There are also portable, lightweight newborn chairs so you can cart them from room to room and get stuff done while they watch.

MATERNITY CLOTHES

Maternity attire emerged in the fourteenth century, when formerly loose and flowy dress styles that accommodated even pregnant figures evolved to be more fitted. It wasn't until the 1990s that maternity silhouettes highlighted instead of hid changing pregnant bodies. And the ready-to-wear styles available now accommodate any size and shape your bump and body take on, any budget or fashion need, and many encourage you to free the bump entirely. From preggings, a.k.a. the stretchy pants you'll be living in for the last months of your pregnancy, to body-con, you no longer have to live with baggy, sister-wife-style patterned dresses or fashion FOMO.

Depending how you carry, your bump might be small at the start of the second trimester, or it might already be poppin', especially if it's not your first pregnancy. That bump is accompanied by bigger breasts, which means your prepregs bra size probably no longer fits. So whether you're showing or still undercover, it's time to find clothes that can comfortably handle these changes.

Most of the hard-core big-belly needs will only be for the last three to four months, so before you binge on maternity clothes, you may be surprised at what you already have, or can get for free. Also, clothing that bears the label "maternity" is often more expensive. A *lot* more expensive. A hack to avoid overpaying is to buy a size up of affordable stretchy options like yoga pants in a normal format. Some other tips:

- Peek into your closet and find the pieces, especially dresses and shirts, that aren't super fitted, or that are stretchy, longer, and have a bit of extra give. Button-down shirts are especially useful, as they work open or closed and can be thrown over dresses. Same with oversize or wrap-style coats for winter months.
- Your breasts are on quite the journey and will expand and contract multiple times in the coming months. Bra extenders are one way to stay in your non-pregnant size as long as possible. Stretchy sports bras are also ideal. And if you do have to buy a larger size, go for a nursing bra so you can use it postpartum.
- Unless your existing T-shirts are long, try bodysuits, as they don't ride up as much. Sure, they can involve more logistics when it's time to pee, but they also look cute over le bump.
- There are plenty of maternity-specific bathing suits, but a normal string bikini is flexible and can last through a pregnancy's many phases.
- For formal occasions, consider renting a dress or rocking body-con or a loose maxi that you can also wear post-pregnancy. When it comes to fancy shoes, choose options with straps and open toes whenever possible and avoid stuffing those poor bloated ankles and feet into tight pumps. Wedges are your friend when it comes to balance in those last months. And if you're wearing a belly band and plan to sport body-con, kinesio tape works well for support and to avoid lines and bunching.

- Interacting with shoes gets progressively harder as pregnancy wears on. Slip-on booties, clogs, and flip-flops will all make your life easier. There are also elastic lace replacements that turn laced shoes into slip-ons.
- Hit up your previously pregnant compatriots to see what they have. Someone you know may be in the middle of a purge, or will let you borrow a few things.
- Speaking of (practically) borrowing, consignment stores, both online and offline, are full of lightly worn maternity clothes—at a major discount. They also often have baby and kids clothes. Score.

Instead of investing too much in a maternity capsule, which you'll want to set on fire by the time you pop, there are also services that allow you to rent clothes during your pregnancy. You can select styles and specific pieces for work, going out, lounging around, or whatever suits your life. They'll ship them out; you'll wear them while they fit and buy any you like; then send the rest back. This is especially useful for formal occasions, like that wedding when you're eight months and feel like a whale, or if your workplace has a dress code.

Hacks aside, there are a few maternity items worth owning. The first and most critical: pants that don't cause pain. There are a multitude of DIY ways to accommodate expanding midsections, by sewing in elastic panels or waistbands to pants you already own. But unless you are really crafty (and dedicated), at some point, you will be forced into the world of maternity pants and/or creative workarounds. And surprise! On the maternity pants front, you may never want to go back, as the proliferation of brands and options are increasingly hip and well cut, and can handle everything from the bloated, I-just-ate-a-burrito phase all the way through your first months postpartum.

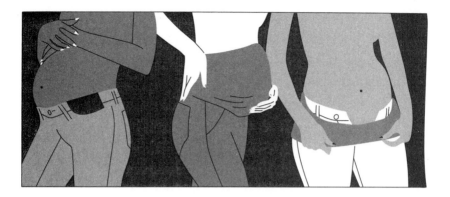

Maternity pants and workarounds fall into a few categories: the under-bump low-rider jeans, the over-bump panel pants, and the I-can't-give-up-my-prepregnancy-pants-just-yet elastic-band hack.

Skirts with elastic waistbands are also useful, from loose maxi styles to more fitted cotton pencil skirts that look a bit more formal. As with many of your prepregnancy stretchy pants, you can push the waistband under or over your bump, depending on which is more comfortable.

You'll also discover the wonders of ruching, the old dressmaker's trick of gathering fabric into pleats so clothes can shrink or expand with one's body. It's a necessary (and — let's be honest — awesome) feature to allow for the growth of your bump in fitted tops and dresses.

To get you started with the basics, here is a suggested list of things you'll actually want to own. Remember that you'll continue to use many of these items postpartum and while breastfeeding (and seriously, you may never want to give up the maternity jeans):

- Maternity pants/jeans and preggings
- Several long-waisted T-shirts
- Sweaters and shirts that layer (your temperature will be all over the place)

- Nursing tanks and shirts that can pull double duty later while you're breastfeeding (get at least one black shirt that won't show breast milk leaks)
- A coat or jacket
- Pj's and loungewear that stretch (darker is better postpartum to hide milk stains)
- A pair of comfortable flat shoes with some extra room (your feet can grow during pregnancy)
- Several non-underwire bras in varying sizes (it's impossible to predict your nursing-bra size, but bonus if they convert)

Okay, now clickhole away!

My maternity wardrobe was mostly loose items I already owned, combined with consignment shop finds and a subscription box service to mix it up for the last four months. I splurged on two pairs of maternity jeans (over-the-bump style), which I loved. My all-time favorite and most complimented purchase was a pair of stretchy black pleather under-bump pants that worked equally well for professional and social occasions, and had the added bonus of making me feel like a superhero.

MEET YOUR PELVIC FLOOR

Going beyond Kegels and
preventing postpartum complications

P regnancy is an endurance sport. No, really—pregnant women have the same metabolic demands as extreme athletes. Unlike ultramarathoners, you are doing the job of growing a human being twenty-four hours a day for 280 days, with no rest days. Which makes it especially important to stretch and find ways to relax and deal with aches and pains as they come.

As we covered earlier, the best advice regarding exercising during pregnancy is: Listen to your body and avoid contact sports. And while staying active is important, it can also be hard. Your body is changing, your energy (like your hormone levels) is all over the place, sleep isn't always great, and staying motivated while you're huge can be a struggle.

Beyond taking a yoga class or a long stroll, there is a body part that you should train that you may not know exists. Or, if you do, you may only associate it with Kegels. However, it's critical to pregnancy and the postpartum period, and neglecting it can cause consequences that last a lifetime.

WTF IS THE PELVIC FLOOR?

Peeing when you sneeze or run might sound like something that happens only when you hit old age, just like the idea of wearing adult diapers. But all bets are off when it comes to the changes in your pelvic floor during and after pregnancy.

If, like most women, you're wondering, *What, precisely, is the pelvic floor?*, it is the set of muscles that support the bladder, bowel, and uterus, forming a bowl shape in your pelvis. They help with everything from bathroom activities to sexual function. A strong pelvic floor is an important part of pregnancy, but also has benefits that last long after, like better sex, more bladder and bowel control, and increased spine stability.

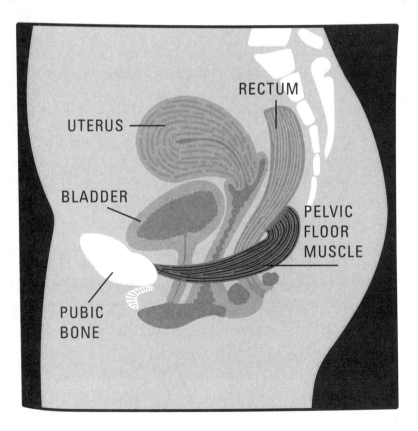

A strong pelvic floor means fewer backaches, a faster recovery after birth, and less postpartum incontinence, one of pregnancy's dark little secrets. Most women assume that incontinence is an inevitability after a vaginal birth, and that there is nothing to be done. Untrue. Also, C-section moms are not immune. Changes to the pelvic floor happen to everyone to some degree because it is stretched to the limit during pregnancy.

A few sample exercises are included below as a gateway to this transformational work. However, working with a pelvic floor therapist starting at around thirty-four weeks through birth, and again six weeks postpartum, also provides tremendous benefit. Starting before thirty-four weeks is also helpful if you feel motivated or are experiencing leakage.

Referrals to a pelvic floor therapist are usually made by a medical provider only if you are experiencing issues like incontinence or pelvic organ prolapse. Few midwives or ob-gyns suggest it proactively. If they do, expect to hear about it during a third-trimester appointment or at your six-week after-birth checkup. But happily, most insurance covers it, and for the low cost of a copay, you can enjoy visits before and after birth remotely or in person. Pelvic floor therapists are usually physical therapists and can help with other postpartum issues like diastasis recti (we'll get there) too. At a minimum, consider going in for an assessment and a one-on-one coaching session to ensure you are doing the movements correctly. This can also be done virtually if you're short on time or if there isn't someone available locally.

AT-HOME PELVIC FLOOR EXERCISES

Consider this your entrée to a stronger, healthier pelvic floor. You may recognize some of these moves from a fitness class or Pilates or yoga, but they take on new meaning during pregnancy.

To perform these exercises, you'll need an elastic resistance band that fits around your thighs, and optionally a yoga mat. It's a ten-minute investment that will pay huge dividends, so try to make it a habit and do them every day.

Do two sets of ten repetitions each, with a thirty-second break between each set.

Bird dogs

- Get in a comfortable position on your hands and knees and flatten your back.
- Engage your abs and straighten one arm out in front of you as you extend the opposite leg behind you, keeping your hips stable and squared to the floor.
- Hold this position for a few counts, then slowly return your hand and knee to the floor, keeping your back flat. Repeat on the other side.

Bridges

- Loop an elastic band around your thighs and lie on your back with your knees bent and your knees and feet hip-width apart.
- Lift your hips up as high as you can, squeezing your glutes while you bridge.
- Relax, lower your hips slowly, and repeat.

Transverse abdominis activation

- Sit on a chair with your feet flat on the floor.
- Contract your pelvic floor like you are doing a Kegel.
- Draw your belly in toward your spine.
- Hold this position for five deep breaths.
- Relax your pelvic floor and abs and repeat.

Clamshell

· Loop an elastic band around your thighs just above your knees.
· Lie on your side on the floor or a yoga mat with your knees out in front of you and bent at a 90-degree angle and your hips stacked vertically on top of each other.
· Keeping your heels together, lift your top knee up to open the clamshell without moving your hips forward or backward.
· Lower your knee and repeat. Then do the other side.

Ride the elevator

· Do not attempt this move with a full bladder.
· While standing or sitting, imagine your pelvic floor at the ground level of a building.
· Contract your pelvic floor, then draw it up through the center of your body like an elevator going up floor by floor.
· After you've contracted fully, hold it for five seconds.
· Slowly send the elevator back down to the ground floor, one floor at a time, then relax and repeat.

PERINEAL MASSAGE

Finally, a little relaxation after all this work! *But wait, my perineum is . . .* Yes, it's the back wall of your vagina, and part of what will later be the birth canal. The goal of perineal massage is to reduce trauma during birth by increasing flexibility and decreasing the resistance of the perineal muscles. Women who do it once or twice a week starting at week thirty-five report less pain at three months postpartum and are less likely to require suturing after a vaginal birth. A pelvic floor therapist or your doula can also walk you through a how-to and may even offer the service during the first stages of labor.

To get started, here are the basics:
- Wash your hands and find a comfortable position (standing, sitting, or lying back) that allows you to access your perineum (after a bath or shower is a great time, as your blood vessels will be dilated, and you're relaxed).
- Apply a small amount of unscented oil, olive oil, or lubricant (no baby oil or Vaseline!) to your thumbs, index, or middle fingers (choose one finger type).
- Insert your fingers an inch into your vagina and gently stretch and massage the back of your perineum by moving your fingers up and down, then side to side slowly.
- Continue to massage for up to five minutes (start slowly and work up to it), reapplying oil as needed.

I gave perineal massage my all and did it from month eight onward. I found the shower to be the easiest massage-parlor location and used olive oil as a lubricant. At first, it was awkward, since reaching anything on your body (much less your perineum) is hard when you're that large, and I had no idea if I was doing it correctly. But after a few sessions (and texts with my doula team), things started to loosen up.

AVOIDING DIASTASIS RECTI

Hold on. During pregnancy my pelvic floor is going to get trashed and now you're telling me my abs are going to split apart too?! What kind of book is this, anyway?

Sorry to be the bearer of bad news, but talk to any friends with kids, and at least a few will complain about their mummy tummy. A terrifying-sounding condition called diastasis recti is the likely culprit.

It happens when the connective tissue in your abdominal muscles weakens and stretches to accommodate your growing baby. This separation can result in the infamous post-pregnancy pooch, or a gap on the linea alba, the fascia that divides your six-pack.

At least 60 percent of pregnant women experience diastasis in varying degrees, and it's not completely preventable even if you follow all this guidance. It happens to nonpregnant people for the same reason — too much pressure on the abdominal muscles. But if you avoid certain activities and moves, your odds of getting diastasis go down, and if you do get it, it may not be as bad. Here are a few tips:

- **Leave the heavy lifting to someone else.** Pregnancy is not the time to become a bodybuilder. Lifting heavy weights or other items more than twenty times per week increases the likelihood you'll develop diastasis. If handling hefty things is a part of your job, talk to your employer. If it happens at home, unless the hefty item is your toddler, leave it to your partner.
- **Avoid crunch-like movements.** Not doing ab workouts while pregnant is intuitive. Taking your time getting out of bed will be, too. The urge to sit straight up may not be. Engaging your abs in crunch-like movements stresses your rectus abdominis.
- **Strengthen your pelvic floor and transverse abdominals.** The earlier you start doing pelvic floor exercises, the better. Building a strong core will help your whole body look and feel better—during and after pregnancy.

One telltale sign of diastasis is abdominal doming or coning when you sit straight up from lying down or move your shoulders off the ground like you're doing a crunch. (But seriously, stop doing crunches!) You won't know for sure until around six weeks after birth, when your provider checks for it.

Diastasis often goes away on its own, and if it doesn't, is treatable, so you aren't stuck with it forever. If you see a pelvic floor therapist, this is a great conversation topic, as they are usually trained to rehabilitate diastasis postpartum and will have tips to help you avoid it.

IT'S NOT A BIRTH *PLAN*— IT'S PREFERENCES

Strategizing and practicing for your ideal birth experience

Some first-time mothers waltz into the labor ward with a list of demands longer than a pop star's concert rider. If you ask a nurse or doctor, there is a correlation between the length of the birth plan and likelihood of a C-section or other complications. If you ask friends with kids, most will tell you that even a textbook vaginal birth has its moments, and that there will be surprises no matter how much you plan.

Though it might seem early, the end of your second trimester is a good time to mentally prepare for labor or your C-section, collect initial thoughts, practice birthing methods, and, perhaps most important, calibrate your expectations. These expectations are often referred to as a birth plan. The word *plan* indicates control, which, as you've hopefully figured out, during pregnancy is not entirely a thing. Even so, feeling in control is a major factor in how satisfied women are with their birth experience. This includes feeling in control of yourself in general, during contractions, and of what practitioners do to you. While pain management might affect your sense of self-control, women who feel that their practitioners listen to and care about them perceive more control over the whole experience. That desire for control spawned the concept of the birth plan.

With all of this in mind, we're going to reframe your desired birth experience as birth *preferences*. There are plenty of ways you can make birth feel right for you, but the most critical aspect is that it ends with a healthy mom and a healthy baby. Also, that the missed expectations, when they happen (and they will in some way), do not make you feel like you failed your transition into parenthood. Your preferences will include things like who you'd like (or not) in the room with you, pain management preferences, and, if all goes smoothly, what you'd like to happen right after birth. We'll refer to birth as *vaginal* or *C-section* and *medicated* or *unmedicated*. Because whether a baby comes out through your vagina or your belly, there is nothing unnatural about your birth, even if it's not what you planned.

Let's pause on this terminology for a moment, as no doubt you've seen the concept of *natural childbirth* floating around. The broadest meaning is that our bodies know what to do during birth and need little or no outside help to do it. Adherents to the purest form of natural childbirth believe that interventions or medications of any kind add risks rather than subtract them, and some are even referred to as "the easy way out." The movement's origin story, however, is not what most people expect.

Grantly Dick-Read is the spiritual founder of the natural childbirth movement, and his work inspired the midwife Ina May Gaskin and many others. As an obstetrician in London in the 1920s, he explored and practiced intervention-free births; a revolutionary idea at a time when procedures like preventive episiotomies and mandatory sedation were common. Dick-Read penned his most well-known book, *Childbirth Without Fear*, in 1942. In it, he claimed that labor pain was psychological, and ultimately due to fear. You read that correctly. He believed that the physical pain women experience during childbirth was all due to their undisciplined minds. The core aim of the book is to cure the underlying cause, the fear-tension-pain cycle, and to make women relax and restore order to their emotions.

Dick-Read's and Gaskin's low-intervention philosophy hits a nerve with everyone today who, rightly, wants to go beyond one-size-fits-no-one hospital birthing experiences. Their message that pregnant women should trust their bodies and themselves is resonant too. The rise of midwifery and doula care also reflect this desire, as both are less interventionist than traditional obstetrics. And less intervention *should* be the goal across every birth setting no matter who is in charge.

However, today's birthing women are older and less healthy on average than those who Dick-Read treated, and there are biological and societal challenges now that did not exist in rural Tennessee at Ina May's famous farm. There are also complications during childbirth—perineal tears, prolapsed umbilical cords, and hemorrhage, among them—that have always existed and often require urgent medical intervention. If giving birth without an epidural or other medication on a birthing ball is your choice and everything is smooth, amazing! But proceeding against a provider's guidance can be dangerous—for you and your baby.

Childbirth is not a contest. Other than safely, there is no right way to birth a baby, no best list of birth preferences, and no gold medal awarded for enduring pain or putting your health at risk. Going without medication does not make you a better parent, just as receiving an epidural doesn't make you a bad one. So shut out the judgment, work together respectfully with your ob-gyn or midwife, ask questions, and choose what is right for you.

PAIN MANAGEMENT

You may already know you'd like to go at it without any medication for as long as you can, and maybe not take any at all. Or you may want to get an epidural as soon as you hit labor and delivery. Maybe you have no clue and just want options. Trying nonmedical approaches first doesn't mean you can't also do the other. A combination of pain management methods is where most people end up—labor earned its name for a reason.

The halo effect of holding a healthy baby right after birth reduces pain and negativity. But unless your threshold for suffering is super-human, even with a prepared mind, at some point during labor, there will be pain. There are nonmedical ways to manage it, like breathwork, meditation, acupuncture, Lamaze, hypnobirthing, and massage. Varying levels of medication outside of an epidural are available for all the different stages of birth, too.

Medication options

The ancient Egyptians wove spells and recited incantations to protect laboring women and unborn babies, and sometimes offered cannabis for pain relief. Made into a paste with apple and honey, it was applied inside and around the opening of the vagina to induce contractions and reduce pain. Opium and folk medicine were other common options until the Scottish doctor James Simpson introduced anesthesia to obstetrics in 1847, first as ether and then chloroform. The tipping point for labor medications came when Dr. John Snow (famed for tracing the cause of one of London's worst cholera outbreaks to a water pump) successfully used chloroform on Queen Victoria during her eighth birth. London's elite quickly followed the queen's lead, and the practice went mainstream.

Twilight sleep, or *Dammerschlaf*, as it was termed by its German inventors, became popular during the suffragette movement seventy years later. Its combination of morphine and scopolamine provided pain relief and had the added "bonus" of erasing the memory of birth altogether. Though American doctors were hesitant to provide this treatment (for good reason, as it resulted in psychotic behavior and nearly comatose newborns), women rose up against what they perceived as oppression and demanded it. Twilight sleep was used for decades until it was replaced by an early version of today's epidural.

Today's labor pain management medications range from what we all know as a standard, catheter-delivered epidural to nitrous oxide. They allow more mobility and more awareness than their previous iterations, too.

The epidural

Over 60 percent of women choose to get an epidural. Women over forty are the least likely to receive one, and those under twenty are the most likely. Go figure. So what is an epidural? It's a type of anesthesia that blocks nerve impulses in the lower back, effectively decreasing feeling in the lower half of your body. The goal isn't to create a total lack of feeling, but rather to minimize painful sensations.

You can receive an epidural anytime during labor, though studies show that starting in early labor can prolong the process or lead to other interventions. Theoretically, you can get an epidural up until the baby starts crowning. The only catch: You need to be able to lie or sit still while it's placed, which can be hard during intense contractions.

There are three ways an epidural can be administered. Your hospital and physician may not offer all of them, so ask about what's possible in a prenatal appointment if you have strong feelings.

- **Standard epidural.** A catheter is inserted into the epidural space in your spinal column and left in place so medication can be dispensed on demand.
- **Spinal block.** A single injection into the spinal fluid, the spinal block works immediately, but lasts only for one or two hours.
- **Combined spinal-epidural.** Commonly known as a walking epidural, it allows more freedom to move around during labor, though it is typically a lower dose and provides less pain relief.

With a standard epidural, an anesthesiologist numbs the area known as the epidural space, which is outside the membrane that surrounds your spinal cord and fluid. A needle is inserted, and a catheter is passed through and taped on for medication delivery. Placing the catheter for an epidural can be uncomfortable but generally doesn't hurt (though the needle does look a little scary). A small amount of medicine will be dispensed as a test to check placement, and, depending on where you are in the labor process, a full dose will be delivered if it is deemed problem-free. The medication itself is a mix of narcotic and local anesthetic to block the pain.

Your blood pressure and the baby's heart rate will be monitored every five minutes to make sure there aren't any changes, and the effects will start ten to twenty minutes after your first dose. Afterward, you can choose to have continuous delivery through the end of labor, or control dosing through a pump that you operate as needed.

Time for upsides and downsides. The biggest upside is obvious—you will have less pain during labor if you get an epidural, though it does not take the pain to zero. As labor progresses, the amount can be adjusted to match where the pain is and how intense it becomes. Today's versions allow you to be awake and alert during labor and birth and may allow you to get more sleep in the early stages as your cervix dilates. Because they are in less pain, many women who receive epidurals claim a more positive birth experience, as they allow more rest.

Now, the downsides. Side effects can include backache, nausea, itching, difficulty urinating, a drop in blood pressure, and in very rare cases a severe headache. They can cause labor to last longer and can lead to interventions like episiotomies and forceps and vacuum deliveries. You will also be hooked up to continuous monitoring for the rest of labor. The lower half of your body may be numb for a few hours after birth, which means you'll be unable to get out of bed and will need a urinary catheter. Though they are less likely to do so today, some physicians and facilities do not allow you to eat after you get an epidural, just in case you need a C-section, which means you'll be on the ice-chip diet until you deliver.

What about the effects on your newborn? Outcomes differ based on the duration of labor and other factors unique to each delivery. Babies born to mothers who chose an epidural had the same Apgar scores as those who didn't. There is also no consensus on epidurals causing difficulty with latching during early breastfeeding. The majority of the medication stays in your epidural space, and little actually enters your bloodstream, so outside of a temporary dip in heart rate, the risks to your baby are minimal.

> *I did not go into labor intending to get an epidural but did not exclude the option. I went through the safety briefing and signed the paperwork when we were admitted just in case. Without giving too much away before the full birth story, after ten hours of back labor, that epidural was the most exquisite pain relief I have ever experienced. It's not without its downsides, but for me, getting an epidural allowed a few hours of sleep during a particularly long, painful, and, as you'll see, complicated labor.*

Nitrous oxide

Used more commonly in Europe than in the US, nitrous oxide is a form of systemic pain relief that is inhaled through a face mask during labor to take the edge off. It provides immediate relief, which stops when you remove the mask. Nitrous doesn't have any detrimental effects on labor progress, and it disappears from your system quickly. However, it is not as effective in managing pain and can cause nausea, vomiting, feelings of detachment, and drowsiness.

Midwives believe the main benefit is relaxing mothers so they don't care about the pain as much, rather than providing true pain relief. Because you are using a mask, it also helps regulate breathing, which can help alleviate anxiety. So if you want to hold off on an epidural and still get some help, this is a safe alternative if it's offered.

> *While I did end up with an epidural after exhausting all other nonmedical options during labor, I started out with a nitrous mask, which I yelled into until I was hoarse. For me, it was more effective as a distraction than as pain relief.*

Narcotics

Administered via IV or injected directly, narcotics, a.k.a. opioids, are used mostly as an alternative to the epidural. Morphine and fentanyl are two of the most common varieties, though different drugs are available pending which hospital you choose. They do not relieve as much pain as an epidural and are not usually given toward the end of labor, as they can temporarily cause neonatal respiratory depression.

Like nitrous, the side effects for you can include nausea, vomiting, breathing problems, and drowsiness. However, as all opioids cross the placenta, there are also some considerations for your baby. Though research is not conclusive, these can range from changes in heart rate and breathing to lower early neurological scores and decreased ability to breastfeed.

Nonmedical pain management

Even if you are planning to use medications at some point, there are methods of relaxation and mindfulness that can help your mind slow down or simply create a more pleasant birthing experience. You can try many of these before birth (some require taking a class or reading a book) and can list your choices on your birth preferences. Techniques range from the commonly known, like meditation and aromatherapy, to those you might not know much about, like Lamaze or hypnobirthing. All of them can provide distraction and more focus during labor and allow you to feel some power over what is happening to your body.

Acupuncture

Though it's believed in Chinese medicine that acupuncture can help stimulate labor, where it has proven results is as a supplement to other pain relief methods during labor. Acupuncture won't shorten labor, but it has been shown to reduce the need for medication. Many women also report a higher level of calm and control when asked about their birth experience later.

A few midwives receive obstetric acupuncture training and certification, so if you have one on your care team, ask if they offer it. Otherwise, some hospitals and birthing centers have acupuncturists on staff, or allow approved external acupuncturists to practice. If you enlist someone from the outside to help during labor or during your pregnancy, make sure they are trained specifically in obstetrical acupuncture.

Aromatherapy

It won't directly decrease pain, but aromatherapy can make the birth experience much more pleasant—for everyone. Powered by essential oils, aromatherapy has been shown to alleviate stress and improve sleep quality in a range of different patients. The benefits also extend to nursing staff, who claim less stress and reduced fatigue and burnout when exposed to calming scents.

Essential oils can be incorporated into a massage, misted on a pillow, or released over time with a diffuser. Labor-recommended oils include lavender and geranium for relaxation; orange, chamomile, and mint for a lift; and clary sage to strengthen contractions. As with all products during pregnancy, make sure the essential oils you choose are of high quality. And before you whip out your diffuser, make sure your hospital or birth center is okay with it in a prenatal appointment. If they are, pack it in your labor bag.

We went into our labor and delivery room fully loaded with lavender essential oil and a white stone diffuser. While it was nice to smell during labor, and essential oils played a role dealing with nausea, it was handiest postpartum. Our room was very popular with the nurses, and felt a bit less sterile.

Hypnobirthing

Hypnobirthing is a mind-body program centered on the idea that fear of childbirth incites tension and physical pain. The goal of hypnobirthing is to relax and avoid going into fight-or-flight mode during labor. The technique utilizes positive thinking, music, affirmations, regulated breathing, and visualization to teach laboring women to self-hypnotize into a calm but aware state. It's thought that the increased sense of calm can help your body release contraction-friendly oxytocin and endorphins, which help blunt pain and make you feel good. Though hypnobirthing is not proven to reduce pain or the number of women who request pain relief during labor, it does confer a sense of control that improves postnatal anxiety and general childbirth-related fears.

If this is a route you want to pursue, involve your partner and anyone else assisting with birth. There are several methods and approaches, which can be learned via an in-person class, or through an app, book, or video.

Lamaze

If you know anything about Lamaze, you likely associate it with staccato "hee hee who, hee hee who"–style huffing and puffing.

Inspired by midwife-led childbirth practices he observed in the Soviet Union in the 1950s, the French obstetrician Dr. Fernand Lamaze created the pattern breathing–focused Lamaze technique to help women relax during labor without medication. It's grown to encompass a more holistic view of the childbirth experience, and centers on six core tenets:

1. Let labor begin on its own.
2. Walk, move around, and change positions throughout labor.
3. Bring a loved one, friend, or doula for continuous support.
4. Avoid interventions that are not medically necessary.
5. Avoid giving birth on your back and follow your body's urges to push.
6. Keep mother and baby together.

The now-international Lamaze organization offers books and in-person and online classes that teach the different methods and framework for coping with pain. As with hypnobirthing, bringing your partner and birth helpers into the training process lets them know how to best support you during labor.

Massage

No need for a professional masseuse—this is a great way to get your partner involved. Massage stimulates endorphin production through tissue manipulation, helps with relaxation, and decreases anxiety. Our body of research is of low quality, but there is some proof that it can provide relief and, at the very least, massage does no harm and is a nice way to bond with your partner.

The gate-control theory of pain is one explanation for why and how massage works during labor. Here's the idea: Non-painful sensations like gentle massage close the nerve "gates" to painful input, preventing pain from traveling to the central nervous system and brain. Because your brain is already busy enjoying the massage, signals from contractions can't interfere and you perceive less pain as a result.

If you're working with a doula, they will share specific techniques in the months before your due date. They'll also be hands-on during birth if you like and can step in to give your partner a break.

Water immersion

Admit it: Labor sounds more appealing when it involves a bathtub and candles. Water immersion doesn't have to mean full-on giving birth in a tub. What it does mean is using water's magical powers to help you relax and temporarily take a load off when labor begins.

Just immersing yourself in a bathtub during the first stage of labor reduces reported pain and the need for medications. The buoyancy helps take some of the stress out of your back and helps create more calming vibes. Not a bath person? Showers are also popular and come with the bonus of being able to point warm water directly at your lower back for pain relief. Some hospitals and birthing centers have a range of both available in their labor and delivery centers, so you can continue to enjoy your tub or shower time even after you leave home.

You may wonder why more people don't just go for it and give birth in a tub. The answer: Depending on whom you ask, the benefits and safety of water births vary. Water births are not for those with complicated pregnancies. They are rarely available at US hospitals, so you may not even have the option unless you want to give birth at home or in a birthing center. There's also the matter of the non-baby "discharge" in the water during birth, which means you might be sitting in poop soup.

Midwives are more pro–water birth than doctors, who are still waiting on concrete evidence before recommending the practice as an alternative to land births. (Yes, that's actually what they call it.)

But whether you're birthing by land or by sea, including hydrotherapy during early labor has no downsides and is a great complement to other relaxation techniques. It may also help reduce the amount of medication you need to manage pain.

Outside of an epic labor playlist created for the occasion, my only passionate birth preference was to spend as much time as I could in the water at home in early labor and later at the hospital as things progressed. This meant that while I was open to an epidural, I chose to delay for as long as I could to retain the ability to bounce between the bed, the yoga ball, and the tub. Remaining active improved the quality of my labor experience and allowed me to feel his progress down the birth canal, which was both incredibly strange and incredibly useful.

TENS machine

More commonly used by our British friends, TENS (transcutaneous electrical nerve stimulation) is yet another weapon in the arsenal of nonmedical pain relief. It sends small pulses of electrical current through your skin into your muscles and tissue, which feels like buzzing or tingling or prickling.

How does TENS help manage labor pain? We don't really know, but assume it's a combination of distraction, endorphin release, anxiety reduction, and preventing pain signals from entering the brain. The TENS device is utilized in early labor, and you can turn it up or down, toggle between different types of pulses, and change the placement based on what you need at different moments. Most of the time, it's used on the back and on acupressure points during contractions.

TENS machines are usually handheld controllers connected to small pads that conduct the current to localized areas like your lower back. For those seeking active laboring options, it's portable—you can clip it to your gown or wear it around your neck, but you'll have to give it a rest if you go into the water. TENS machines are not a standard feature of hospital birthing suites, sadly—the most likely people on your care team to have a TENS machine are doulas and midwives.

I'm not sure how effective the TENS machine was in relieving pain, but I did like the way it felt. Sort of like a pleasant, very low-grade electrical shock. I found it most useful for spot treatment on the lower back and, while on full blast, as a distraction from the peak of contractions.

NEWBORN CARE AND PROCEDURES AFTER BIRTH

Now that you've thought about your preferences during labor, it's time to think about what happens right after your baby is born. Many of the options below are just that—options. As far as your baby goes, as you'll read, there are few downsides to the suggested protocols. Though, as with everything, it's your decision.

Delayed cord clamping

The umbilical cord, the connection between the placenta and your tiny bundle, follows the baby out during delivery, right before the placenta makes its farewell. Most of the time, the cord is immediately clamped and cut within seconds of birth. With delayed cord clamping, there is no severing of that connection for several minutes, or until the cord stops pumping. Some people choose to level up further by milking, or by squeezing the cord several times after it stops pulsing, to infuse the infant with all possible blood.

So what are these benefits? Most studies have been done only in preterm infants, but these babies have higher iron levels, concentrations of hemoglobin, delivery room temperatures, blood pressure, and urine output.

How about risks? To date, there has not been enough research to prove that past concerns like jaundice or postpartum hemorrhage are valid. But most studies have been done in homogenous populations, so we don't fully understand whether there are nuances with more diverse ethnic backgrounds.

You cannot delay cord clamping if there are complications during birth for you or the baby. It's also sometimes not possible during a C-section birth, though you can ask.

Cord blood banking

Umbilical cord fluid is loaded with stem cells, which can be used to treat immune, genetic, and neurological diseases like cancer, leukemia, and anemia. Cord blood contains ten times more stem cells than bone marrow, rarely carries any infectious diseases, and is half as likely as adult stem cells to be rejected. The collection process is painless and takes only a few minutes. Before cutting the umbilical cord, officially separating mom and baby, the doctor clamps it, inserts a needle, and collects a minimum of 40 milliliters of blood. The cord blood is then sent to a lab or bank to be tested and stored.

Where it goes to be stored is up to you. Public cord banks make donated cord blood available to anyone, including researchers, and don't charge for storage. Private cord banks store for your family's use only, but charge processing and storage fees, which are in the thousands of dollars.

So is it worth it? If you're doing it for insurance against future issues, probably not. The odds that your child will use cord blood are low, and it may be good for only fifteen years. Private banks are recommended only if there is a sibling with a medical condition who could benefit from it, or a family history of leukemia, lymphoma, sickle cell anemia, or other rare genetic disorders. However, if you'd like to contribute to research, or help build the supply, public banks are a free way to give back.

If you decide, *Yes, I want this,* cord blood banking requires advance planning. Talk to your practitioner between twenty-eight and thirty-four weeks so they can put you in touch with organizations that work where you are giving birth, and ensure they have a collection process available. Four to six weeks before you're due, get in touch with a bank to coordinate the pickup.

One other consideration: If you decide to delay cord clamping, it's not always possible to bank cord blood, as most of the blood in the placenta and umbilical cord will go into your newborn's body or begin to clot. Public cord banks have minimum donation requirements, so the smaller amount may not qualify. Family banking typically imposes smaller volume limits and can be fine even if you delay. If you'd like to attempt both, just talk to your practitioner.

Placentophagy

Let's talk about the practice of consuming your placenta after birth, or the custom's official name, placentophagy. A reminder: The placenta is an organ that grows in your uterus exclusively during pregnancy to act as a gateway between you and the baby. The placenta transmits oxygen and nutrients and removes waste from your baby's blood through the umbilical cord, synthesizes hormones, and is partially to blame for your increased estrogen and progesterone levels. It is expelled from your body in the first minutes after birth, as its mission of sustaining your baby during pregnancy is accomplished.

If placentophagy is a new concept for you, perhaps you are thinking, *Um, okay, why would I want to eat one of my own organs?* Many mammals eat their placentas, whether to remove the scent and by-products of birth to avoid predators or for reasons we don't yet understand. While placenta is a longtime ingredient in Chinese medicine, the first recorded instance of placentophagy in the US was documented in 1970, in a young woman living on a commune.

Now, on to the science—or lack thereof. There are very few placentophagy studies, done with humans or animals, and there are zero done with any real gold-standard rigor. The only one that holds to that standard was a pilot study involving twenty-three women that found no significant differences in maternal iron status post–placenta consumption versus a beef placebo.

There are also risks. The first is related to how the placenta is stored and processed. It can contain an accumulation of potentially harmful substances, like Streptococcus agalactiae, which is a major cause of neonatal sepsis. Using placenta to prevent postpartum depression leads many women to delay getting the medical and supportive care they need, too. There is also no evidence that eating your placenta actually has any preventive or positive effect on postpartum depression.

Long story short, the dearth of research means that we do not fully understand the known risks, that the advocacy is without physiologic basis in fact or science, and that nearly all the information out there is purely anecdotal.

If you plan to pursue placentophagy, do so with caution and find a reputable practitioner. If you are working with a doula, it may be a service they provide.

Hepatitis B vaccine

At birth, there is just one vaccine that will be offered for your baby—hepatitis B. There is no downside to getting it out of the way, but some pediatricians are willing to do it at an early well-child visit. If this is your preference, indicate it on your birth preferences.

Eye drops

Another post-birth protocol is the squirt of the antibiotic eye ointment erythromycin to prevent eye infections in newborns. If you give birth in a hospital, it is mandatory in most states. The only side effect (and it's rare) is eye irritation.

Why is it important? When the baby passes through the vagina, they can be exposed to bacteria and pathogens that lead to infection, and sometimes blindness. The most common perpetrators are STDs, especially gonorrhea and chlamydia. Before you say, *But there is zero chance I have an STD! Do I still have to do it?*, there are other types of bacteria like E. coli found down there, and the drops protect against that, too.

If you'd like to delay the drops until after golden-hour bonding and breastfeeding, that's fine.

Vitamin K shot

Newborns depart the womb with low levels of vitamin K in their bodies. Vitamin K helps blood clot, so if levels are too low, it can cause dangerous bleeding in the brain or intestines. It's hard to come by in breast milk, and babies don't typically get good access to vitamin K until they start eating solid foods at around six months.

This single injection eliminates that risk; there are no side effects, and there's no compelling reason not to do it. As with the eye drops, waiting until after you've had that first bonding session to administer the shot is just fine.

Circumcision

Circumcision is the surgical removal of the penis's foreskin, the natural extension of the skin of the penis. On the inside, foreskin is more like the inside of your mouth or eyelids and secretes a natural lubricant. It contains blood vessels, neurons, skin, and a mucous membrane that covers and protects the glans, or tip of the penis. The foreskin's exact biological purpose and whether it should be kept intact depend entirely on whom you ask. Answers range from "a worthless flap of skin whose role as protector was replaced by boxers and briefs" to "critical as a shield for the sensitive glans and full of nerve endings that increase sexual pleasure."

Circumcision is the most practiced surgical procedure in human history. Its origins can be traced back to ancient religious and coming-of-age rituals, and it is still practiced in the Muslim and Jewish faiths. Roughly 33 percent of the world's male population is circumcised, and about two-thirds of those are Muslim. In the US, it rose in popularity during the Victorian era to prevent masturbation, but now only a little over half of adult males have the procedure performed, and that number is dropping. It is even less common in Europe—20 percent across the continent and just under 4 percent in the United Kingdom.

Today's version takes just a few minutes and costs about $300. In a typical circumcision, the baby receives a topical anesthetic or numbing agent; then the foreskin is clamped or separated by a plastic bell from the glans to cut off the blood supply. The surgeon then uses a scalpel to remove the foreskin and dresses the wound. Healing time is seven to ten days, and complications are minimal, just 0.4 percent in infants. That rate rises to 2 percent for older children and adults, so if you're leaning toward yes, it is better performed on newborns.

So why do it? Outside of religion, the most frequently cited reason parents circumcise is so that father and son match. Major medical organizations endorse it for the public health benefits, as epidemiological studies in sub-Saharan Africa have shown that the risk of contracting HIV drops 50 to 60 percent for circumcised heterosexual males, and 30 percent for other sexually transmitted diseases like herpes, HPV, and syphilis. We don't really understand why, and these numbers do not directly translate to all populations. Other health benefits include fewer urinary tract infections (UTIs), a reduction in penile cancer, and better overall cleanliness. The long-held concern that circumcised men are not able to feel as much as uncut men may not be true either. Though it's difficult to prove definitively, one review shows that there is no difference in sexual pleasure or sensation attributable to circumcision status.

There are also reasons to question whether circumcision is worth it. The number of UTIs in infants is very low, penile cancer is rare, and benefits related to STD transmission all but disappear with condom use. When it comes to pleasure, there are studies that show increased sensitivity during sex in uncut men, and more pleasure for their partners with the added friction of the foreskin. Some parents opt out because they feel it's not their decision to make, that their child should decide for themselves later. Others believe the procedure is traumatizing (though it's not clear if a newborn remembers it) and that if a child was born with a foreskin, unless it's for religious reasons, there's no reason to remove it unless it's causing harm.

Like so many other decisions related to pregnancy and raising kids with no clear-cut (sorry!) answer, this one is up to you and your partner to make.

Rooming-in versus nursery

Gone are the days of you and your first post-birth guests gazing over a field of incubators and brand-new babies behind glass. As part of new baby-friendly practices, many hospitals are shifting from a communal nursery to rooming-in, which means your baby will hang out in your room with you after birth. Some hospitals are doing away with nurseries entirely as a cost-cutting measure, which is another reason it's so important to do a pre-birth tour and understand what to expect.

Whether you have a vaginal birth or C-section, there are challenges to recovering from both. And while rooming-in or not doesn't have to go into your birth preferences, it can, and regardless is a good thing to understand before you arrive in your postpartum room. Know that the nursery is an option even if the hospital follows baby-friendly practices, assuming they still have one. In that scenario, the baby is brought to you from the nursery for feeding, or you can walk down. The default is to leave the baby with you to encourage breastfeeding and bonding in those early days.

Sorry, data junkies—current research does not support or refute improved rates of exclusive breastfeeding with rooming-in, as sleep is an important input into milk supply, as is the frequency of feeding in those early days. There just aren't enough high-quality studies yet. So if you find yourself exhausted and need a break for a few hours, ask for it. It is your right. If you are at a baby-friendly hospital that no longer has a nursery, ask your partner to take the baby for a stroll around the postpartum ward.

PUTTING IT ALL TOGETHER

The final list of birth preferences captures whom you'd like to have in the room (also anyone you don't), laboring and medication preferences, what you'd like to happen after birth, and newborn care, assuming all goes smoothly. As with wit, brevity is the soul of a good list, so try to keep it to one page, and use bullets and bold anything important so it's easy for your care team to scan. Remember, these preferences can all go out the window as labor progresses, so try not to be wedded to any one thing.

The following outlines the big decisions for a hospital or birth center delivery and includes contingency plans in case decisions need to happen on the fly. Print out a few copies so you have them on hand for different shifts (hospital providers usually rotate every twelve hours, at 7:00 a.m. and 7:00 p.m.), and in case any copies become casualties of the labor process. Take it to a prenatal appointment midway through the third trimester to discuss with your ob-gyn or midwife, as it's important they be able to accommodate your choices.

Brief introduction to you and your partner, and any other birth team members

- Have fun with it, be polite, and give them a sense of your personality since when you hand it over, you won't quite be yourself.
- Include phone numbers for your support team and your baby's pediatrician.
- If there is anyone you don't want present, list their names, too.

Quick overview of obstetrical and medical history

- Number of pregnancies and births with delivery method
- List of medications, allergies, and chronic conditions

Personal/setting the mood

- Would you like to bring music? Any lighting preferences if available?
- Do you want to labor and give birth in your own clothes?
- Whom would you like in the room during birth (partner, doula, family, etc.)?

Medical and labor preferences for vaginal delivery

- Would you like monitoring (continuous fetal monitoring, etc.)?
- Do you want pain medication during labor and delivery? If so, which (nitrous oxide, epidural, etc.)?
- If you're unsure, would you like a saline lock (a flexible tube placed in your arm or hand that can deliver IV medications) placed?
- If you're at a teaching hospital, are you okay with medical students participating in your birth? (Resident participation is usually nonnegotiable.)
- Whom would you like to cut the cord?
- Would you like to delay all nonessential newborn procedures until after skin-to-skin?

Medical preferences for cesarean delivery

- Whom would you like to be present in the OR?
- Would you like to hear the details of the procedure as they happen and have the surgical drape dropped so you can see the baby during birth?

- Do you want the cord milked?
- Do you want to hold the baby or do cheek-to-cheek immediately after birth (if possible)?
- Do you want to breastfeed within the first hour?
- Do you want your partner to do skin-to-skin if you can't?
- Do you want to delay newborn procedures until after skin-to-skin (if possible)?

Baby

- Vitamin K shot, eye drops, hepatitis B vaccine
- Bath timing (at hospital or delay until you go home)
- Circumcision (if applicable)
- If neonatal care in the NICU is required, whom would you like to be there?

Postpartum

- Breastfeed or formula feed?
- Rooming-in or nursery?
- Other requests related to pain management, stool-softener/laxative preferences, preserving your placenta

To give you an example of what birth preferences can look like, here are mine. My answers may not be your answers (there are no right answers—these were just my preferences). Some people get really creative and make it visual, others are much longer, some are briefer. The only nonnegotiable is to ensure it reflects you and your desired experience.

Birth preferences for Schrock,
(soon-to-be) party of three 🎉 🎉 🎉

Meet our team

Mom: Leslie (writer, strength-training fan, chocolate-chip cookie enthusiast)
Dad: Nick (code name "Nickipedia," for encyclopedic knowledge
   of world history)
Doulas: Meleah & Heather

The medical stuff

Please do not discuss/offer pain medication during this vulnerable time.
If I'm feeling discouraged, please support me with positive affirmations and
general encouragement. I will ask for nitrous or an epidural if needed
but would like to remain unmedicated for as long as possible to have
an active labor. **NO MISO** and **NO FENTANYL**

Second stage of labor

Please allow me to position myself for comfort (all fours, squatting,
side-lying, standing, etc.).

In the event of a cesarean birth

- Nick and doula present in the OR the entire time
- Music
- Delayed cord clamping and milking the cord
- My baby to stay with me through recovery
- Full skin-to-skin contact in the OR
- All newborn procedures delayed until I have had the chance
  to bond and breastfeed

We look forward to a wonderful birth and thank you for your support.

Second-Trimester Checklist

☐ Finalize childcare decisions for the months after birth and your return to work.

☐ Learn about and create a draft of your birth preferences.

☐ Book a tour of your birth center.

☐ Sign up for birth class.

☐ Speak to your employer about family leave benefits (partners should do this, too).

☐ Enjoy a surge of energy and reprieve from some of your pregnancy symptoms (hopefully)!

☐ Start to put together the nursery.

The Third Trimester

The home stretch! As the weeks wear on, your walk will become a waddle (try swinging your hips to combat this tendency), the extra weight in front (and constantly shifting baby) means your balance will be different every day, and sleep will become increasingly difficult. You may even be able to see the outline of a foot kicking or a tiny fist trying to punch its way out. While this starts off as a novelty and never stops being an amazing (if strange) feeling, when your baby is jammed up into your ribs toward the end, it can also be very uncomfortable. This discomfort also comes in the form of abdominal spasms caused by hiccups in the middle of the night, and a tiny head pressing down insistently on your bladder.

Speaking of tiny body parts and discomfort, the third trimester is when your doctor or midwife will start talking about kick counts. Though it doesn't have to involve a swift jab to the ribs, movement is an easy way to monitor well-being over time. The reason it's important: Studies show maternal detection of kick counts can help predict adverse outcomes, as changes to a fetus's movement patterns can indicate stress or other problems. The best way to measure your kick counts is to have a tall glass of water and a snack, then lie down on your left side or back, take note of the time, and count the baby's movements. You'll want to do this during a time they are usually active and count each kick until you get to ten. Make a note of how long it took in your phone or on a piece of paper and do it every day around the same time to keep tabs.

This is also the time to mentally and physically prepare to meet your baby and understand what happens during birth. But don't forget, you're going home after it's all over. If you need support immediately afterward, it's good to get this lined up as soon as possible.

Let's not forget about your recovery either. Baking and birthing a human is hard work, and your body will need a little extra love postpartum. Putting finishing touches on the nursery is important, but so is having a few items on hand to make you feel good.

When I had to size up from a 32D to a 34E bra, I worried that my boobs were actually growing around my body and would soon connect in the back.

As I rolled into the third trimester, I looked pregnant enough that people no longer hesitated to say congratulations, ask how far along I was, or touch my bump. I was fine with friends doing it impulsively but found this behavior by strangers mystifying. My bump was of the straight-out torpedo variety, which apparently made it a very tempting target. One woman said rubbing a pregnant belly (while rubbing mine) is considered good luck, which didn't really make me feel any better, or lucky. So I learned to politely tell people who attempted to touch that I wasn't interested. After all, no one ever rubbed my stomach when I wasn't pregnant!

SO WHAT'S HAPPENING IN THERE?

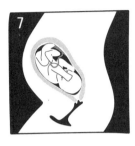 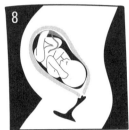 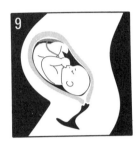

Month 7

Baby: Starting in week twenty-eight, your baby will be a little over two pounds and measure around fifteen inches long. Most growth and development from now on will be in the brain (making connections) and packing on fat. The fat not only is helpful for temperature regulation once they join the outside world; it also means their skin will no longer be transparent. Patterns of sleeping and waking are more consistent moving forward, which means there will be an increasingly noticeable rhythm to fetal movement. By the end of the month, they will be over three pounds and sixteen inches long, getting close to their final birth length.

You: If you think the second trimester was crazy for growth, you ain't seen nothing yet. Strap in—your body is in for some major changes. Expect stretching, more pressure in your pelvis, and a decline back into first trimester–style fatigue as your abdomen continues to expand. Fun fact reminder: The distance between your pubic bone and the top of your uterus in centimeters corresponds to the number of weeks you are. This measurement is called the fundal height and is more accurate the later into a pregnancy you are. Your baby still has room to scoot around, which you can probably feel at times, but by the end of the month may get comfortable in a head-down position. Your dreams can intensify and feel more real, even though your sleep quality may decline. Try to focus anxious energy on what you can get done and less on everything you imagine might go wrong during birth.

Month 8

Baby: Entering the ring at three to four pounds is your baby in month eight. And while they may be a flyweight for now, after packing on around a half pound per week, they'll end the month between five and six pounds and eighteen inches long. The main items on the agenda this month are practicing the basics of sucking, breathing, and — as you'll probably feel more and more frequently in your ribs with more baby and less amniotic fluid as a cushion — kicking and stretching.

You: Pop! That's the sound of your belly button, which may start protruding this month. As the space in your abdomen gets more crowded, you may become a bit more breathless as your uterus will start to crowd your lungs until the baby drops farther into your pelvis in preparation for birth. Trips to the bathroom may become increasingly long and/or complicated as digestion will continue to be sluggish, causing constipation and hemorrhoids. But one bathroom activity is here to give your poor pregnant body a break. Spend twenty minutes in the bathtub to give yourself a little reprieve from gravity.

Month 9

Baby: In the final month before their debut, your baby is packing on around half a pound per week, ending up somewhere between six and ten pounds, and measuring between nineteen and twenty-two inches. The last-minute preparations to emerge involve readying their systems for launch, building their brains, and shedding the vernix, a.k.a. that cheese-like skin coating. The cramped quarters mean that there may not be quite as much fetal movement in these final weeks, but you should still watch out for any changes in activity.

You: It's almost over. Finally. You may not even notice pregnancy symptoms at this point, as you've had nine months to get used to them. Weight gain may level off, but expect vaginal discharge to pick up, your digestive tract to misbehave in all the ways you've grown accustomed to, and, once the baby's head drops, your runs to the loo to be more frequent at all times of the day and night. Braxton Hicks contractions, also known as practice contractions, may be constant in the last weeks.

Third-trimester symptoms and solutions

Braxton Hicks contractions

- When does it happen?
  Can happen mid–second trimester but are most common in the third

- Symptoms
  Tightness in abdomen, usually after exercise or sex

- Cause
  Unknown but believed to help tone the uterine muscle and help blood flow to the placenta

- Solutions
  Hydrate, and change positions. If they become painful or regular, or don't stop when you change position, call your physician, as they could be a sign of preterm labor.

Carpal tunnel syndrome

- **When does it happen?**
  Can happen in the second or third trimester and persist postpartum

- **Symptoms**
  Pain, tingling, or numbness in your hands

- **Cause**
  A form of edema, or built-up fluid, in your wrists that squeezes your median nerve

- **Solutions**
  Treat with hand splints or ice, or use cabbage leaves as cold compresses around your wrists, acupuncture, or stretching exercises.

Depression

- **When does it happen?**
  Though there is more focus on postpartum depression, it can start anytime during pregnancy.

- **Symptoms**
  Loss of interest in activities you used to love, decreased ability to feel pleasure, feelings of worthlessness, fear, guilt, or suicidal thoughts

- **Cause**
  Hormonal swings, changes in your body, the major life changes happening

- **Solutions**
  Speak to a loved one, schedule an appointment with your doctor, contact a mental health professional, or call a hotline.

Restless legs syndrome

- When does it happen?

  Can happen anytime during pregnancy, but can pick up in the third trimester, especially at night

- Symptoms

  Tingly or crawling sensation in your leg or foot while you are sitting or lying down that prevents you from feeling settled

- Cause

  Root cause is unknown, but genetic factors are suspected. Can also be triggered by iron, magnesium, or vitamin D deficiency.

- Solutions

  Avoid caffeine late in the day.

Edema

- When does it happen?

  Seventy-five percent of women experience some edema or swelling during pregnancy, though it tends to be worse toward the end of the third trimester.

- Symptoms

  Swelling and fluid retention in your ankles, hands, and feet

- Cause

  Can happen in warm weather, or after too much time sitting or standing up; like stretch marks, edema is largely genetic.

- Solutions

  Take plenty of breaks throughout the day to move, and put your feet up when you are sitting, limit your salt intake, choose comfortable shoes, and try compression socks or stockings.

Sciatica

- When does it happen?

  Can happen in the second trimester, but is more common as your body gets bigger

- Symptoms

  Sharp or shooting pain in one or both sides of your butt or leg, numbness, difficulty walking, standing, sitting, or generally doing anything else

- Cause

  Muscle tension and increasingly unstable joints triggered by relaxin and your expanding pelvis, the weight of the baby on your sciatic nerve

- Solutions

  Stretching or non-weight-bearing exercise like swimming. If you need the big guns, physical therapy, acupuncture, massage, or chiropractic care.

FOR PARTNERS

If you peeked at the above third-trimester symptoms, you'll know that outside of a rapidly expanding midsection, mom-to-be will be tired and moving more slowly, especially in the final weeks. Ways you can add major value: Head up final preparations to welcome the baby home, give your partner a massage, and help put together a postpartum kit for her, too.

You may be feeling anxiety around the birth, which is totally normal. That's why the chapter on birth is here—so you both have an idea of what to expect. Make time to talk to your partner about how she would like to be supported during that experience. Your role can vary from chief labor cheerleader to running interference with family or providing a hand to squeeze.

Prepare for the baby

Going shopping isn't always fun (for either of you, especially in the last weeks of pregnancy), but creating a space that is well outfitted and safe is much easier before you return home with a newborn. Though you may not care about nursery color schemes or diaper brands, whether by doing something as simple as making sure everything is assembled or taking charge of online ordering, find a way to be engaged. You'll be a hero, and the process of putting together your baby's soon-to-be space will make it feel more real for you, too.

Be her advocate—and keep an eye on her health

This is especially important right around labor, as she will be exhausted, you know, about to eject a tiny human from her body. If you didn't help put the birth preferences together, now is an excellent time to get familiar with them. Understand exactly what she wants if everything goes well, and what to do if things go not quite as planned. If she is concerned about pain management, or really doesn't want a C-section, make sure that you are talking to your practitioners and understand the rationale for each decision.

Most critically, start watching her health. If you see her struggling, ignoring health symptoms that could indicate something more serious could be happening, or observe anything else that feels out of character, talk to her. The cadence of prenatal appointments picks up toward the end of pregnancy, and her provider will take her blood pressure and track other health metrics. But it's also a good idea to have a blood pressure cuff at home, as she'll spend far more time there than at a doctor's office.

LIFE RIGHT BEFORE—
AND AFTER—BIRTH

Preparing for your baby's arrival, packing your hospital bag, planning parental leave and childcare—and living with a newborn

There is no way to sugarcoat this one: The final weeks of pregnancy can be rough.

Many women feel a late hit of energy and an urge to nest and clean. Others find themselves panicking about what will happen during birth. Still others wonder when or if their baby is ever coming out. And combined with the logistics of coordinating leave, it probably feels like the list of things you should be doing is endless.

Birth is treated a lot like a wedding. The focus is so heavily weighted toward THE BIG DAY that we neglect to think about the big picture. Just like waking up the morning after your wedding with a marriage to maintain, after birth, a tiny human will exist outside your body with needs you must fufill for the next eighteen years. Maybe longer if they move into your basement. Not to mention, you must manage your own physical recovery. The third trimester is your time to mentally and physically prepare for birth and, just as important, what happens when your baby is a part of your daily life.

BIRTH CLASS

Around month six, as your bump looms larger and the kicks grow more vigorous, birth becomes less abstract. And that can be scary. But chances are, you're not the only anxious party. The idea of standing by and watching someone push a human out of their body is difficult for most people to visualize and can end with your partner fainting if they are not mentally prepared.

Since your partner hasn't had an active physical role in pregnancy outside of moral support, foot rubs, and food fetching since their initial contribution, birth class is a great opportunity for you to bond and deal with the growing reality. And bonus: The education will give them the tools to be a great birth coach.

All hospitals and birth centers have different classes on offer, ranging from marathon sessions in a single day to shorter classes that stretch out over weeks. If a doula is helping with your birth, sometimes they are willing to teach a class privately if your schedule is less flexible. And there are destination childbirth classes taught at resorts if you want to earn extra credit during your babymoon.

Classes usually happen in a group setting, with moms and supporters showing up to learn together. They are taught by midwives, physicians, nurses, and doulas. The goal of birth class is to provide a solid foundation that allows you to make educated choices regarding your care. The curriculum covers everything from interventions like fetal monitoring and the circumstances in which you may need to have an unexpected C-section, to decisions regarding pain management, and ways to relax. For those who haven't seen a live birth, they will show video footage so you are mentally prepared. Don't worry, it's less gory than you might expect, and you'll marvel at the power of the female body (and how wide that cervix can stretch!). Other classes are very hands-on and teach breathing and massage methods.

Go with a smaller class size if you can and think about how you best absorb information. If you are a hands-on learner, make sure an experiential portion is part of the package. More of a visual or aural learner? Watching videos and listening to lectures may be the way to go.

The benefits of these classes go beyond education. Like group-based prenatal care, they're also a way to make new parent friends. Nothing like going through the trenches together, right? This is especially useful if you'd like to pool childcare resources, or don't have many friends with kids and are seeking potential playgroups. Welcoming a child is a big change, and being around other new parents provides huge emotional benefits.

Even if this isn't your first childbirth rodeo, the landscape and options change quickly, so signing up for a refresher isn't a bad idea. And if you're really into studying and learning, childbirth class is just the beginning. There are breastfeeding lectures, pain management classes led by anaesthesiologists, infant CPR and first-aid courses, and classes on specialty methodologies like hypnobirthing too.

TAKE A TOUR AND PREREGISTER YOUR STAY

Whether you plan to deliver at a hospital or birthing center, labor is not the best time to get the lay of the land. Take a pre-birth tour of the facility so you know where to go and exactly what to bring. Partners, you can use this visit as an opportunity to scope out food availability so you know what to pack for yourself, and see what your sleeping situation entails.

Outside of identifying things like the entrance and parking, here are a few questions you may want to ask on your tour:

- Will I labor and deliver in the same room?
- Are rooms private or shared?
- Is there a place for my partner to sleep in my room?
- Do you offer rooming-in so my baby can stay with me after birth? Does the facility have a nursery if I need rest?

- How long is the typical stay for a vaginal delivery? What about a C-section?
- What are your visitor policies and hours?

Many facilities allow you to preregister your stay for birth, reducing the need to fill out paperwork between contractions. Others don't require it. You may be able to do this on the tour, or after one of your prenatal visits, so just ask your ob-gyn or midwife. You'll still need to show an insurance card and ID when you check in, but preregistering will get you into the hands of your care team more quickly.

PACK YOUR BAG

Plenty of people arrive at labor and delivery with nothing but clothes for their trip home and rely on the hospital to provide the rest. The only can't-give-birth-without-them items are your ID, your insurance card (if you have one), and that infant-friendly car seat. That said, consider packing a few things to help you feel human in the aftermath.

The restorative power of the first shower after birth is unreal, so at a minimum, bring items that the hospital doesn't provide—toiletries like shampoo, soap, a toothbrush, and toothpaste, and real clothes for your departure—and call it a day. The bonus of hospital gowns is that you don't have to wash them. But getting into some of your own comfortable clothes is nice too.

Depending on where you give birth and their policies, there is room to be creative, which you may have indicated in your birth preferences. Some moms rock out to a labor playlist using a portable speaker in a room that smells like lavender thanks to the diffuser they brought from home. Others bring their full complement of getting-ready items to help them feel more like themselves post-birth, and dress in their own cute labor-compliant gowns to avoid the open-back, butt-out hospital variety.

There is no right list, only what makes you comfortable as you welcome your new tiny human. Think of it as packing for a two-to-three-day trip if you are planning to give birth vaginally, and three to four with a C-section. Favorite products or clothes may still be in circulation during those final weeks, so make a list on your phone of anything you aren't packing now and print it or text it to your partner so you both remember what's missing when it's time to go.

As a place to start, here is a mom- and labor nurse–approved list of suggestions and bonus items:

For mom

- Insurance card and ID (must have!)
- Two physical copies of birth preferences
- Comfortable clothing (bring washable versions as they may not make it through birth and early breastfeeding unscathed)
  - Loose-fitting items like yoga pants, pajamas, and nursing tops for pre- and post-birth
  - Cotton robe
  - Dark bottoms, loose top, and comfortable shoes for the ride home
  - Warm socks and/or slippers (socks need grippy bottoms—yoga or Pilates socks work well)
  - Flip-flops to wear in the shower
  - Big, comfortable postpartum underwear (if you don't want to rely on the hospital's mesh panties and giant pads)
- Eye mask and earplugs (hospitals are loud and every nap counts)
- Travel-size toiletries (shampoo, conditioner, soap, toothbrush, toothpaste)
- Hairbrush (hair dryer if you want to feel fancy)

- Beauty products (like moisturizer, body lotion, cleansing wipes, dry shampoo, and lip balm)
- Entertainment (book, tablet, portable speaker)
- Phone charger (with a long cord, as outlets are usually far from the bed)
- Snacks
- Pillow and towels (hospital varieties are thin)
- Aromatherapy diffuser and essential oils (optional but makes the stay more pleasant)
- Toilet paper (bathroom activities are stressful enough postpartum and the hospital's scratchy stuff is unpleasant)
- Gifts for awesome nurses (snacks or treats are great)

For partner

- Two wardrobe changes
- Warm hoodie or sweater
- Pajamas (or anything comfy to sleep in)
- Slippers or slip-on shoes
- Toiletries
- Entertainment (book, tablet, laptop)
- Phone charger (with extension cord)
- Sleeping bag (see what bedding the hospital or center provides while on your tour, but the standard foldout couch isn't comfortable)
- Folder to collect all the paperwork you'll accumulate

For baby

- Infant car seat
- Mix of clothing and accessories for photos (going-home outfit is most crucial)

- Nursing pillow (if you plan to breastfeed, especially if you are planning a C-section)

So what did I take? Answer: most of the things on this list. Friends told me about the mystical first after-birth shower, and I knew from my hospital tour that none of the accoutrements I wanted were part of the stay. Yes, I was that person with the essential oil diffuser, a small portable speaker (and multiple playlists for different moods), my favorite toiletry items, and a few inexpensive but cute hospital-like gowns for before and after. Though I shed them after a few hours of labor, it was nice to have something reasonable to put on during recovery. The item I was most relieved to have was nice toilet paper, as bathroom visits are scary for a while (especially the first poop), and hospital toilet paper is the worst.

CHOOSE A PEDIATRICIAN

Just like prenatal care, there are a range of practitioner options for your baby's medical needs. From hospital-based physicians to doctors who run progressive private practices and will come to your home, you have plenty of choices to suit your priorities and needs.

Pediatricians are the most popular choice for infants, and, like any other medical subspecialists, they are trained to handle the specific health conditions and milestones related to tiny, growing bodies. Establishing an early relationship with a pediatrician sets the groundwork for up to twenty-one years of your child's life, as many pediatricians work from infancy all the way through adulthood. They provide preventive care, make sure growth and development are on track, and act as primary-care physicians.

It's difficult to find good online ratings and reviews for doctors, and much of what one person dislikes or loves is personal preference. You might care about their education and years in practice, philosophy on breastfeeding or sleep training, which hospital you would visit in an emergency, how they handle triaging patients to other providers when they are not available, or how they feel about prescribing antibiotics. How much time you get in each appointment is a hot-button parent issue. Each practice operates differently, and the individual slots can be as short as fifteen minutes or as long as an hour.

Many practices offer getting-to-know-you visits and interview opportunities so you can get a sense of your prospective physician's approach and personality. You may want to introduce yourself to the other partners at the practice, as over the years you will see more than one of them. If you are torn about where to start, just choose one and try a few visits when your baby joins the world to see how the physician interacts with them. You can always change later.

REGISTER FOR A BREAST PUMP

Early human breast pumps were based on technology used in the dairy industry. The first breast pump patent was filed in 1854 by Orwell H. Needham. In his application, he describes a pump bellows connected to a nipple shield that women could press to release the flow of milk. Over the next century, other similar cow-inspired models hit the market, mostly to help infants who had difficulty nursing, or if a mother had inverted nipples. Then, in 1991, today's market leader, Medela, introduced the first consumer-grade electric breast pump, and the industry took off.

If you plan to breastfeed, with fairly minimal effort, you can save the $200+ you might have spent on a breast pump, as private insurers, Medicaid, and even some hospitals will provide or lend them to you at no cost. Your insurer works with outside vendors to manage medical devices including breast pumps, so your first step is calling for that information. Next, you'll visit these vendor websites (which are named things like Yummy Mummy) to see what's available. There should be a wide variety of brands and styles.

So how do you choose? If you are a frequent traveler, or will be pumping at work, features like "battery-powered" and "readily available replacement parts" are critical. Noise is a concern if you plan to pump in the same room with a sleeping baby or partner, or at work.

One detail that should be mandatory in all electric pumps is the ability to toggle between stimulation and letdown modes. Stimulation does what you would assume—stimulates the flow of milk. After about two minutes, you'll manually or automatically switch into letdown or expression mode, which is designed to maximize that flow.

Looking for something more portable? There are a growing number of wearable pumps that nix the wires and bottles in favor of small, self-contained, rechargeable units that nestle into your nursing bra. They are quiet and discreet enough that you can walk around, take a call, or go out to lunch—all while pumping. Convenience and aesthetics aside, wearable versions are generally not as powerful as corded pumps, so it may take a few extra minutes to finish each session.

The only other major thing to figure out when purchasing a breast pump is the circumference of your nipple so that you order the correct-size flange. The flange is the cone-shaped pump part that seals directly onto your breast. If it doesn't fit correctly, the suction won't work, so it's important to get it right. This may take several tries, as tissue elasticity can also affect sizing. Most pumps come standard with a twenty-four- (the size of a quarter) or twenty-seven-millimeter flange by default, so if you need something bigger or smaller, check with the manufacturer to make sure they make that size before you place your order.

If your pump arrives pre-birth, go through the sterilization and setup and play with it. There are a lot of parts to sort through and clean, and it's not always clear how it fits back together. Buy a few breast-pumping bras as well, so you can go fully hands-free even with a corded unit. Most pumping bras don't require exact measurements, just a size range, like sports or lounge bras, so you'll be fine selecting one in advance. If you'd rather skip the electronics, there are hand-expression pumps available as well.

One of the benefits of writing this book was having an excuse to try out all the pumps. So I got one of each—corded, hand, and shove-it-in-your-bra-and-walk-around.

The hand pump was retired quickly, as other than building up my hand strength, it was too much work to use often. But it was useful as a backup, and good to put on during breastfeeding to catch drips from whichever breast was not in use.

The corded version was the most powerful and fastest on full throttle. If I had to pump when I was particularly full, or in a rush, I always used it. But it was heavy, it had many parts, and when I did use batteries, the suction was much weaker, and they drained within a few days.

The wearable pump was amazing, though not quite as un-obtrusive as it purported to be. But it was much quieter than the corded version, and allowed me to do most things, including video and conference calls, without thinking much about the fact that I was also pumping. The only downside: It took me a while to figure out the latch, and I made a mess taking it off, then getting the milk into bottles. But it was perfect for on-the-go, as it had fewer parts to clean and was much lighter.

CHOOSE YOUR BABY'S NAME

Though odds are this process (or negotiation, as it is for many couples) started months ago, it's time to get serious about whittling down your options. If you did not choose to learn the gender in advance, this involves agreeing on two different names so that no matter which way it goes, you're covered.

Some parents go into birth with a few names they like and wait until they meet their child. Others have a family name picked out before they're even pregnant. Whatever your jam, it's a permanent decision, which can feel like a lot of pressure. However, if you ask most parents later, they can't imagine any other name for their child once they give it.

You don't have to know the name the moment your baby is born, though if you are in a hospital, choosing before you are discharged means it can go on the birth certificate and flow into all associated paperwork with less hassle. If you decide to go home without naming your baby, you'll have to coordinate with your State Department of Health, which is about as fun as it sounds, and adds cost. If you're giving birth at home or in a birthing center, you'll also need to get in touch with them to fill out a birth certificate.

Still riffling through books and scanning websites or need a way to trim down the options? Here are a few thoughts from the parent hive mind:

Naming pro tips

- Look at and say the full name together to make sure it flows. Same goes for initials, and making sure they don't spell anything questionable.

- Think about possible nicknames, especially for a long or formal name. Kids' personalities don't always match.

- Same with obscenities, rhymes, and famous associations. If you don't think of them, their friends at school will later.

- Have a name you love? Everyone will have an opinion, so it's up to you to decide whether to share. If you do, be prepared to stand by your choice.

You are likely to be regaled with commentary from people who have an ex, a family member, or a frenemy with the same moniker.

- If you choose a unique spelling of a common name, know that it will be misspelled most of the time.
- Right now, you are naming a baby. But your baby will spend most of their life as an adult, so be sure the name ages well.
- If you and your partner can't agree, and you plan to have more than one child, flip a coin, and take turns.

PARENTAL LEAVE

If you work and anticipate going back, you'll need to plan. And it's the last thing you'll want to deal with during your final weeks of pregnancy. Start this process a few months before your due date. This goes for you too, partners. Paperwork to add your new family member to a health insurance plan needs to be filled out in advance too. If it's not outlined in your company benefits, call your insurance provider for specifics. The typical timeline is thirty to sixty days after birth to add your baby to a policy.

Below is a list of advice that applies to both of you:

Two months before birth

- Document everything so your daily duties and responsibilities at work are easy for others to access and understand.
- Start training your coworkers or replacement.
- Check in with your boss on your return-to-work timeline and set expectations around how available you will be while out of the office.

- Stop by HR and fill out any required paperwork related to leave or internal policies.
- Put together a preliminary childcare plan so you don't have to scramble in the post-birth haze while you are recovering. Day care centers in large cities often have long wait lists, and you'll want to visit before you enroll your baby.
- Explore breastfeeding policies and find out where the pumping room (if it exists) is in relation to your workspace. If there is no pumping room, ask your manager what other accommodations are available.
- Talk to other parents who have taken leave. Ask for their advice, any regrets, and things you may not have considered.

Right before you leave

- Remind coworkers how often you'll be available for questions, and when you will return to the office.
- If you plan to breastfeed, block time on your calendar after your return for pumping (thirty minutes at a time, three times per day). It's easy to remove from your calendar, but harder to make time when you are getting back into things.
- Set out-of-office email and voicemail reminders.
- If you plan to shut off entirely, turn off push notifications and deactivate your email inbox on your phone so you don't get any messages.

CHILDCARE

It can feel overwhelming (also sad) planning caregiving for a baby you haven't even met. But because timelines and wait lists are long, and it's the single most expensive out-of-pocket cost for the first few years of your baby's life, it takes a lot of advance planning. Finding the right childcare setup takes time, research, and budgeting.

If you'd like help at home during your first months postpartum, the time to find that person is at least three months before your due date. Infants are allowed in most day care centers as early as six weeks, so if you need coverage before that time, you'll need a nanny or helpful family member or friend. There are also rules governing childcare centers and nannies that differ by state to understand, depending on which you deem best. No matter which you choose, the top criteria should be quality and safety.

Day care

Many day care centers, especially in cities, have wait lists that span months or even years, so start exploring options as early as you can.

Pros

- Generally the most affordable option
- Set hours and calendar so there is less chance of a schedule interruption, and gives you plenty of time to plan for closures
- More transparency regarding their operations via online reviews and state regulations that ensure they are safe, compared with private caregivers
- Socialization with a larger group of babies at an early age

Cons

- Most accept only full-time applicants.
- Schedule has no flexibility.
- More germs mean higher likelihood of kids getting sick, which means you'll need backup childcare or to take time off
- Less one-on-one time from a caregiver

- Pickup and drop-off are less convenient than someone coming to your house.

Family childcare centers

Smaller centers that operate in someone's home are a more intimate day care option. Standards differ by state, but most require a license to care for children that aren't relatives unless they meet specific criteria or provide only occasional care. Licensed centers are monitored to ensure they meet health and safety requirements, and that the caregiver receives training (CPR/first aid) and passes a criminal background check. You may be surprised to find one or more of these centers in your neighborhood, as they aren't always obvious or don't have a sign out front. Some specialize in infant care, while others have mixed age groups.

Pros

- Price is usually lower than larger day care centers.
- Fewer children than a day care, and mixed age groups provide a family-like environment with younger and older children as well as siblings.
- More flexibility on schedule than a typical day care, and some offer overnight services.
- Home environment is more personal than a day care.
- Closer relationships with providers, since there are usually only one or two.

Cons

- Your child will be in a person's home, not a facility designed specifically for babies and children, so a safety assessment is important.
- If the caregiver or caregiver's child is ill, there is often no backup person and the center will be closed.

- Schedule is less predictable, as that caregiver's schedule and life will impact closures.
- If you or your child doesn't jive with the primary caregiver, there are no options to change classrooms.
- Finding one is often via word of mouth and requires more research, as many don't advertise. Read reviews and ask for referrals.

Nanny share

A nanny share is somewhere between a family childcare center and a full-time nanny. It is great for parents who need more flexibility and is less expensive than having a full-time nanny as your employee. A nanny share is hosted in either your home or another family's and costs run around one-third less than a full-time nanny's hourly rate. It's a guaranteed way for your baby to get one-on-one time and socialization with another early friend, too, and a way for you to build your network of fellow new parent friends.

Pros

- More personalized care
- Early friendship and bonding for your baby
- Flexible schedule in case your needs change (depending on the other family's needs)
- Nanny may be available for overnights and weekends

Cons

- Costs are higher than day care and include benefits like paid vacation, sick leave, and holidays, and you'll pay nanny taxes.
- There will be more management and paperwork, as the nanny is technically an employee.
- If you share hosting with the other family, each of you will have to buy extra supplies for each location

Nanny

Having a full-time caregiver at your disposal is great for parents who need flexibility, work nonstandard hours, or travel. It is the most personalized childcare option, as there are newborn specialists with multiple certifications, career nannies who speak multiple languages and cook, and those who offer flexible part-time help. If you're considering a nanny, think about the traits that matter most to you, and whether there are other aspects like cultural background that you'd like your child to experience. Be thoughtful about what personality type will best suit your whole family, as this person will spend a lot of time in your house.

For a nanny or nanny share, it can be hard to book someone far in advance the way you would day care, so start looking three months before you need them, as they'll have a better sense of their availability. The only exception to this timeline is newborn specialists, as they can book up as early as the first trimester. There are sites with candidates you can search, nanny placement agencies, and local mom groups with referrals. Before you commit to a candidate, do reference checks. If you're hiring someone after you give birth, do an in-home test to see how they are with your baby. Hearing them say they know how to give an infant a bottle is different from seeing them do it. Open communication is critical to a good caregiver relationship—on both ends. It can be nerve-racking to leave your child with a new person, especially in those first months. Trust is everything.

Pros

- More personalized one-on-one care for your child
- Flexible schedule in case your needs change (although be reasonable—they have lives too)
- Ability to choose someone who has skills like teaching your baby another language or driving, to be able to take them to activities like swim lessons

- A nanny's primary job is childcare and other needs related to your baby (like laundry, food preparation, bottle cleaning, etc.), but some are willing to help with household tasks and errands. Discuss this during the interview process, as some are willing to pitch in and others require more pay to do additional work.

Cons

- There will be more management and paperwork, as a nanny is legally your employee.
- Costs are typically around three times that of day care and benefits usually include paid time off (holidays, vacation, and sick time) and sometimes healthcare and other perks.
- When your nanny is sick, you will need to find a backup person or drop-in option, or you will have no childcare.
- It is hard for some parents to watch their baby bond with and sometimes prefer another person. The one-on-one relationship between a nanny and a parent can also be complex and is why trust and communication are so critical.

Au pair

Au pairs are caregivers in their late teens or early twenties who exchange childcare and other household services for room and board and a stipend. Usually, they travel from a foreign country to live with a host family for six to twelve months. They can introduce your baby to their culture, language, and they become part of your family during their stay.

The au pair option won't work for a newborn, as au pairs are not legally allowed to take care of infants under three months of age. But they are cheaper than nannies and have the added benefit of living in, which enables a wider range of possible hours.

Pros

- Hugely flexible since they live in your home
- Less expensive than a nanny
- They typically speak another language, so your child can benefit from bilingual immersion.

Cons

- Au pairs are only legally allowed to work a maximum of ten hours per day and forty-five hours per week and must have one and a half consecutive days off per week. If your needs go beyond that, you'll need supplemental childcare.
- Space—an au pair needs a separate room in your house to live in.
- They will be with you for one or two years at most, so it's not a long-term solution unless you are comfortable rotating through different people.

Staying at home

Some parents who plan to return to work do the math on childcare costs and realize they are close to (or in excess of) what they would bring home. For others, leaving their infant in the hands of a care-giver proves too hard. Some decide to take a break when their kids are young and return to work when their youngest starts kindergarten. Combined, these factors mean that even if you have every intention of going back to a full-time job after birth, sometimes it doesn't happen immediately. And it's no longer just moms who are staying home—18 percent of stay-at-home parents are now dads.

Pros

- You get to bond with your baby one-on-one as the primary caregiver.

- No effort spent sourcing or managing outside help
- Full control of your baby's schedule and exposures to different classes and experiences

Cons

- If you plan to return to work later, there are long-term impacts on your salary and career.
- It can get lonely and isolating, and stay-at-home parenting requires building a strong support network of other parents.

POSTPARTUM PREP KIT

Hospital bag? Check. Email auto response ready to go? Check. Baby name? (Maybe) check. Frozen maxi pads and mesh panties? Huh?

If you give birth vaginally, you'll have discomfort down there for a while. C-sections have a different set of struggles but also require extra recovery care, especially the incision. If you don't want to buy now, you can snag some of these items from generous nurses before you check out of the hospital, so make friends and ask for extras.

Must-haves for everyone

- Overnight and heavy maxi pads
- Loose-fitting underwear (stock up on hospital mesh panties, and buy your own disposables)
- Compression wrap or belly binder (helps to hold everything together while your organs return to their original locations—ask the hospital for one)
- Stool softener
- Large water bottle
- Nipple ointment or lanolin (even if you're not breastfeeding, your nipples will be sore)
- Blood pressure cuff (your doctor may prescribe one

if you have hypertension or other conditions, but it is valuable to have one on hand postpartum)

Vaginal births

- Frozen-padsicle ingredients (alcohol-free witch hazel, aloe vera, spray bottle) or perineal spray
- Medicated cooling pads (Tucks or similar)
- Sitz-bath soak
- Peri, a.k.a. perineal irrigation bottle (yes, watering your perineum after birth is a thing)
- Donut pillow (especially if there was tearing)

C-sections

- High-waisted underwear (to minimize the band rubbing against your incision)
- Breastfeeding pillow (to keep the baby's weight off your abdomen)
- Vitamin E and silicone sheeting for scar treatment once your incision closes

There is one other piece of equipment that you should consider having on hand for the postpartum period, and that is useful for the final months of pregnancy especially if you are constipated: a defecation posture modification device, a.k.a. poop stool. It helps to decrease straining and increase bowel emptiness even when you're not pregnant. The first postpartum poop (and those in the weeks after, especially if you had a C-section or any tearing) can be terrifying. Coupled with high-quality toilet paper, a simple stool that turns your sit into a squat can fend off the bathroom scaries.

THE BIG EVENT

What really happens during birth

Like a tiny tropical storm gathering strength, your baby is finally ready to make landfall. What transpires during birth is influenced by whether it's your first pregnancy, the position of your baby, how you'd like to labor, medication choices, and where you choose to deliver. Also, biology! Vaginal birth is unpredictable and can start anytime. Scheduled C-sections are usually done at around thirty-nine weeks.

Whether you watched too many medical dramas or heard horror story after horror story from friends or strangers online, it's normal to be nervous about the unknowns (and pain) of labor. Same goes for a C-section. Enough women fear pregnancy and childbirth that there is a clinical term for it—*tokophobia*. While it may not feel that way while you're in it, the memory of labor pain during vaginal birth is short-lived.

Hopefully, building your birth preferences will help you feel confident asking questions when you need clarification or want to understand why a treatment was suggested. This applies to medical staff and anyone else managing your care, as ultimately, it's your job to weigh the risks and benefits and self-advocate. Informed consent, meaning you and your provider talk and make decisions together, is at the heart of these relationships. If you can't shake the anxiety or feel unable to manage by yourself, consider getting a doula or ensure that a partner or friend you trust is ready to be by your side.

With that, here is the science of childbirth in all its glory, and how vaginal and C-section births work.

One small (huge?) birth fear story.

At our thirty-two-week ultrasound, my son was measuring 58 percent for overall size, but his head was already over thirty-five weeks(!!!). No surprise there, as Nick's is also giant. This revelation reinforced my number one birth phobia: tearing. When it came time to discuss birth-related concerns with our doula, she reminded me that that area is meant for stretching, and suggested I visualize his head flying out of my body while saying or thinking the phrase "My vagina is HUGE!!!" Though I am not really an affirmations person, "My vagina is HUGE!!!" became my internal rallying cry every time I felt anxious.

I get that the idea of not remembering or being able to describe labor pain sounds unbelievable. I didn't believe it before birth either. But even a week afterward I had flashes but could not actually articulate it other than to say labor hurt. I suspect the memory lapse is nature's way of ensuring we do it more than once.

VAGINAL BIRTH

Your baby's arrival has been marked on your calendar for close to a year, and if your due date is approaching, the flood of texts and calls to check in has probably already begun. Unfortunately, unless you have an induction or C-section scheduled, there is little chance that day will be their actual birthday, as (reminder!) only 5 percent of spontaneous vaginal births happen on the projected due date. Sixty-six percent occur within seven days, but the way we calculate gestational age just isn't very precise.

It's best to look at your due date as a range, not a guarantee. Most practitioners stick with dating from your last menstrual period, but not everyone ovulates on cycle day fourteen, not all cycles are twenty-eight days, and not every embryo docks in the uterus on the same schedule. There's also human error to factor in, as it's easy to forget or misreport your LMP. Another factor: genetics and family history. If your mother, sister, or mother-in-law had a long pregnancy, so, too, could you.

But what about those third-trimester ultrasound measurements (if you have them)? Wouldn't those be more exact? We touched on this before, but no. In the first months of pregnancy, babies are about the same size regardless of how large they grow to be at birth, which is why they map closely to LMP. In the final months, measurements and dating are based on an average that just isn't accurate for some larger babies. Trying to estimate weight toward the end can also be surprisingly imprecise and off by one or two pounds.

For first-time mothers, the estimated due date may actually be three to five days after forty weeks, and there is no difference in pregnancy duration based on the baby's gender. Fifty percent of first-time mothers will go into labor on their own by forty weeks and five days, and 75 percent will give birth by forty-one weeks and two days. If you are coordinating your birth and postpartum support, give them a date with a week on either end. Same for parental leave, as planning to wind things down professionally by forty weeks ensures you won't be fielding emails on your way to labor and delivery.

The last few weeks of pregnancy are an important developmental period for your baby, so though you may be ready to eject them from your uterus after such a long stay (and, of course, you're excited to meet them), don't rush too much. You can't put them back in once they come out.

Into the breech

Some babies have a hard time finding the exit. About 3 to 4 percent of pregnancies end in what's known as a breech birth, where instead of arriving at the cervix headfirst, the baby has its butt or legs pointed down. Even if yours is slow to make moves, that means that by term, 96 to 97 percent pull it off even if they wait until the last second.

Breech babies are usually detected halfway through the third trimester, which provides time to try to turn them before they are full term. One relatively low-risk (but painful) method to correct it is called external cephalic version (ECV). It's been around since the days of Aristotle and involves manually turning the baby around at thirty-six or thirty-seven weeks. An ECV always happens in a hospital just in case it causes premature labor or bleeding. A doctor or midwife applies firm pressure and gently turns the baby up and away from the pelvis. Some women find it just slightly uncomfortable; others describe it as excruciating as labor, which is why an epidural is sometimes offered. ECV works 60 to 75 percent of the time, and once the baby is pointed in the right direction, it has less than a 5 percent chance of going breech again before birth. But not everyone can try it. Carrying multiples, previous C-sections, low levels of amniotic fluid, large babies, placenta previa, and other pregnancy complications exclude you. If you're weighing whether or not to do it, ask your provider for their ECV success rates.

If ECV isn't for you, or doesn't work, there are fetal positioning and spinning methodologies that suggest different movements and exercises. Acupuncture and chiropractic care are two alternative avenues along with playing music near the pelvis. And if you like water, spending time floating in a pool belly down sometimes entices a baby to flip.

If breech presentation can't be fixed before birth, most providers recommend a C-section. Though one hundred years ago vaginal breech birth used to be managed by midwives, most ob-gyns and today's midwives feel the risks outweigh the benefit, or their hospital may not allow it. Many are not trained to perform them either.

Attempting to give birth vaginally with a baby in the breech position is dangerous and a common cause of infant mortality.

Vaginal breech birth complications can include cord prolapse (the cord comes out of the cervix before the baby), head entrapment, and if there is pressure on the cord or it gets pinched, it can decrease the flow of blood and oxygen to the baby. Simply put, the risks of a vaginal breech birth are higher for you and your baby than a C-section.

Are we there yet?

Sorry, there is no way to coax a baby out of your belly before they're ready. While there is little definitive evidence on the below methods, they won't do any harm and give you a way to pass the time.

- **Go for a walk or climb stairs.** Hills and inclines are less painful if you have pressure in your back, as is walking on softer surfaces like grass or a track. Coupled with a little fresh air, the exercise may also help you be less stir-crazy in the final weeks.
- **Sex.** Not only are these last weeks your final opportunity for intimacy sans baby, but the female orgasm also does double duty and releases oxytocin, which is the main ingredient in Pitocin, the most common medication used to induce labor. Semen is also high in prostaglandins, which help to ripen the cervix.
- **Nipple stimulation.** Before trying this route, run it by your ob-gyn or midwife, as it can be powerful. If they say yes, it's exactly what it sounds like, and you can do it manually or with a breast pump.
- **Acupuncture or acupressure.** Research is limited, but the hypothesis is that acupuncture stimulates the uterus via hormonal changes or the nervous system. It is most effective when your cervix is already at least partially open for business, so make sure you coordinate timing with your provider.

- **Eat dates.** Several studies have shown that eating six to eight Deglet Noor or three to four Medjool dates daily starting in week thirty-six helped women have higher rates of spontaneous delivery, shorter labor, and less need for induction. It's thought that they help ripen the cervix. More is not better, so don't eat a whole bag. Even if it doesn't work, dates are packed with fiber, which helps with constipation.
- **Membrane sweep.** You'll need some help for this one. Also known as membrane stripping or a cervical sweep, it can bring on labor if you are nearing an induction or late. Your provider will put a finger into your cervix and with a circular motion separate the amniotic sac from the cervix and stimulate prostaglandins. It can be uncomfortable and painful and cause spotting, and there is a risk of a ruptured amniotic sac (premature rupture of membranes, when your water breaks but no labor is happening). You may go into labor within hours, or it may be that nothing happens.

The siren song of internet ads or products promising a "natural" way to induce labor can be very tempting. But beware, as some products can do harm. Before using any teas, oils, or herbs claiming results, talk to your ob-gyn or midwife about the side effects.

When forty weeks came and went with no action, I took long wad-dles to the park, marched up and down the stairs, used an electric pump to stimulate my nipples, had giant pregnant sex, doubled my date consumption (hey, I was constipated), and had two different membrane sweeps. The membrane sweep might be the one thing I'd skip if I had it to do over, as it was incredibly painful and did not achieve its intended effect.

Induction

Labor induction can happen for a variety of reasons: preeclampsia, gestational diabetes, premature rupture of membranes, not enough amniotic fluid, chorioamnionitis (a uterine infection), and other medical conditions. The most common reason it's done is if pregnancies last beyond the due date.

Most ob-gyns encourage induction by forty-one weeks if labor hasn't started on its own. If you hit the forty-two-week mark, the placenta may not be able to support the nutritional needs of your baby, and there is an increased risk of stillbirth. The ARRIVE study (A Randomized Trial of Induction Versus Expectant Management) showed that healthy first-time mothers who were electively induced between thirty-nine weeks and thirty-nine weeks, four days, were less likely to need a C-section. It is not standard protocol, and it is not offered at every hospital, but your ob-gyn may ask if you're interested. Most physicians still recommend letting nature take its course unless there is a reason not to.

The Bishop score is a calculation providers use to predict how close you are to labor, and whether an induction is likely to work. The score combines changes to your cervix—position, dilation, effacement, and the consistency—with the position of the baby's head. Seventy-five percent of first-time mothers who are induced go on to have a successful vaginal delivery, which means one in four still end up with a C-section. Depending how far along things are, you may experience one of several induction routes.

The first is to ripen your cervix using prostaglandins or a Foley or bulb catheter. The Foley is a small balloon that is gradually inflated to dilate the cervix manually. Another method is an amniotomy, which involves physically rupturing the amniotic sac with a small hook. This is done only if the baby is well positioned, and the cervix is partially dilated and effaced. The most well-known induction tool is Pitocin, a synthetic version of oxytocin, the hormone that causes the uterus to contract. Pitocin is not used to ripen the cervix, so you won't receive it until things are a bit further along. It usually makes labor contractions more intense and can shorten the breaks between.

Induction does have risks. Oxytocin and prostaglandins can over-stimulate the uterus, decreasing blood flow through the placenta, which can then lower your baby's heart rate. The powerful contractions can also rupture scars from a prior C-section or other uterine surgery. And there can be more bleeding after delivery, as sometimes your uterine muscles get fatigued and then don't contract when you need them to. Most ob-gyns won't suggest it if you have placenta previa, a breech baby, umbilical cord prolapse, active genital herpes, or any other condition that would be unsafe for the two of you.

Signs labor is imminent

The insane truth is, we have no idea exactly what triggers labor. Hypotheses include that babies are born right before they will no longer be able to navigate the narrow human pelvis on the way out, or that a chemical produced in the baby's lungs alerts the mother that they are now capable of breathing on their own, and that the length of a pregnancy is limited by the mother's metabolism. Whatever the trigger, and hopefully researchers will put some muscle behind finding the answer, there are well-established symptoms that tell you labor is imminent.

Braxton Hicks versus real contractions

You may feel these practice contractions throughout the third trimester, but closer to birth the frequency will increase. So what is the difference? Braxton Hicks contractions, known as false labor, will cause your uterus to harden, but moving or changing positions usually makes them stop. Real contractions are like a moving train. They don't stop and get more intense and frequent over time. True labor can render you speechless, which is a sign to head to labor and delivery.

Baby drops

For first-time moms, the baby drops farther into the pelvis two to four weeks before labor starts. "Lightening," as it is also called, can also happen at the start of labor. The good news: Breathing will be easier now that your baby isn't pressing on your lungs. The bad news: Your baby will now be exerting pressure on your bladder, which will multiply your round trips to the bathroom.

Cervical ch-ch-changes

Think of your cervix like a turtleneck. It stretches and thins to accommodate the baby during birth, then returns to its original size. Cervical changes are key to birth, and one of the first signs of labor your practitioner will look for is cervical dilation or opening. It begins at one centimeter and, by the time your baby's head is peeking out, will grow to ten centimeters.

But birth is not just about cervical dilation. For your baby to exit successfully, cervical dilation *and* effacement need to happen. Cervical effacement, or ripening, is the thinning of the cervix. During labor, your cervix shortens and pulls up and becomes part of the uterine wall. Effacement is measured as a percentage, and, like dilation, can also happen slowly in the weeks before labor, or more suddenly during labor itself.

Diarrhea

Though your stomach may get squirrelly anytime during pregnancy, diarrhea is more likely to happen in the weeks and days before labor starts. Why? Because of chemicals called prostaglandins and because, alas, your rectum, like the muscles in the rest of your body, is relaxing to prepare for birth. Keep a bathroom within easy waddling distance.

Weight loss or stabilization

The increase in bathroom breaks coupled with lower levels of amniotic fluid may mean your weight gain stops, and that you even drop a few pounds in the final weeks of your pregnancy. Have no fear—this has nothing to do with your baby's health.

Bloody show and mucus plug

Though it sounds like a horror movie, the appearance of the bloody show and mucus plug are happy signs you'll meet your baby soon. The opening of your cervix is blocked throughout pregnancy by a mucus plug, designed to keep bacteria and other bad stuff out. Imagine draining a bathtub: When your baby is ready to make their appearance, the plug will come out, pre-labor, accompanied by thick discharge. Spotting is normal, but if you experience heavy bleeding, call your practitioner immediately. There is no need to store and carry your mucus plug to labor and delivery or text a picture of it to your practitioner. They've seen hundreds, and unless there is something really weird happening, they all look about the same.

Water breaks

While rom-coms would have you believe that it happens as a gush in the produce section, usually your water breaking is much less dramatic. Sometimes it's a trickle of amniotic fluid. Occasionally, it's a very watery surprise. Other times, it happens in the middle of the night as you're sleeping.

When it happens, your first move should be to call your provider. In 8 to 10 percent of pregnancies, water breaks before labor without contractions. This is called premature rupture of the membranes (PROM) and though labor hasn't officially started, it may mean an induction is imminent. Why? Because a ruptured amniotic sac is at risk for infection if labor takes too long to kick off.

Contractions or not, contact your care team when your water breaks to check in. If you feel that whoosh and it's green or brown, that could mean meconium (your baby's first bowel movement) in the amniotic fluid, which can be dangerous if swallowed by your baby. Bright red is another sign you should see someone immediately. And if your water broke and twenty-four hours come and go with no real contractions, head to labor and delivery anyway.

THE STAGES OF LABOR

Stage 1

Early labor

Early labor is the longest and mildest phase of labor. It can last anywhere from six to twenty-four hours (sometimes longer) and will end with your cervix three or four centimeters dilated. If you're wondering if you are actually in labor, just remember the phrase "longer, stronger, closer together" and apply it to your contractions. It's one way you can tell a contraction is the real thing versus Braxton Hicks. The other is that moving around or drinking water won't make contractions go away—they will remain intense for thirty to forty-five seconds.

Since it takes a while to kick into active labor, and most hospitals will not admit you until you are in it, it's time to get comfortable at home. Distractions designed to keep you relaxed and your anxiety at a minimum are key during these early hours. Achy back? A warm shower or heating pad is a great solution. Most physicians suggest avoiding the tub at home after your water breaks to avoid infection, since your baby is no longer protected by the fluid-filled sac, so wait for your warm bath until you go to the hospital.

Though it may sound unavoidable, don't forget to pee. A full bladder can slow labor from progressing. If you're hungry, now is not the time to scarf down a pizza or huge meal. Have a light snack. Once contractions are less than five minutes apart, it's time to go to the hospital or birth center.

Now to the inevitable question: What does labor pain feel like? It is categorized in two ways: visceral pain and somatic pain.

Visceral pain comes during the initial stages of labor and is described as internal pain—dull or aching, squeezing, and sometimes sickening, as it can be accompanied by nausea and vomiting. It can feel vague and diffuse, as it's not typically confined to one area. During phase one of labor, the uterus pushes the baby against the cervix so it dilates in order to move them through the vagina. Most women compare it to intense menstrual cramps.

Somatic pain comes once the vagina stretches and opens, beginning late in early labor and continuing through active labor. It is much more intense, localized, and easier to pinpoint, and is described as a sharp or burning feeling as the pelvic floor, perineum, and vagina stretch and distend, and uterine contractions intensify.

If your next question is *When will I know when it's time to leave the house?*, the answer is in that phrase "longer, stronger, closer together." The 5-1-1 rule is an easy way to remember—you should have a strong contraction every five minutes, each contraction should last for one minute, and this rhythm should happen for at least one hour before you bolt.

Active labor

Congratulations, your cervix graduated from three to four centimeters dilated and will soon be closer to seven. Active labor takes an average of eight hours but could take up to eighteen. Oof. By now you'll likely be in the hospital or birthing center (if you're not, it's time to go!), and whoever is there to coach and support you will be fully engaged.

Your attention will be focused on the rise and fall of contractions by now, so if you haven't already, pull out the labor coping and relaxation methods you've been practicing so you can preserve your energy and try to stay calm. If you did not get an epidural, walking around or trying different positions or a warm bath is a good distraction. If you're in the thick of it and feel like you need more pain management, now is a good time to ask for that, too. Get some rest before the final stage (if you can).

The use of perineal warm packs during this stage of labor can prevent third- and fourth-degree tearing, and reduce the instances of urinary incontinence at twelve months. If you are working with a doula, this is something she may do. If not, nurses and partners are good candidates for this job.

Transitional labor

So named because it is a transition from labor to pushing, transitional labor is the shortest and most challenging phase, taking between thirty minutes and four hours. Your cervix dilates from seven centimeters to ten, and contractions will last between one and two minutes with a thirty-second to two-minute rest between.

Transitional labor is tough, so lean on your support person as much as you can—literally and figuratively. It's not always pretty, either. Symptoms you may run into include chills and hot flashes, nausea and vomiting, and other forms of gastric distress.

Stage 2

Pushing

Fire up the hip-hop—it's time to push it. Your cervix is fully dilated at ten centimeters, and you will start to feel an intense urge to push. The pushing phase can last from twenty minutes to three hours, depending on how the baby is positioned. Contractions will be forty-five to ninety seconds, with three to five minutes of rest in between. Take every moment of rest you can and use a mirror to check things out if you need extra encouragement or just want to watch your baby enter the world.

The best part of this phase is that it ends with the first glimpse of your baby's head crowning. That feeling, while magical, can also involve a lot of burning or stinging (there's a reason the crowning effect earned it the nickname "the ring of fire"), as your vagina and perineum are stretching to their limits. When the baby starts crowning, your provider may tell you not to push anymore. Controlling the rate of the head crowning is how your ob-gyn or midwife prevents tears. They may also apply warm compresses to your perineum for the same reason. Warning, if you're using a mirror to monitor progress, the head can slip in and out. It doesn't mean your labor is stalling—just stay focused and listen to your coaches.

There may be poop. Yes, the rumors are true—though it doesn't happen to everyone, many women pee and/or poop during this phase of birth. Mentally prepare yourself and your partner that it's not only normal but common, and one of the many reasons the beds in labor and delivery rooms have waterproof covers. The medical staff is well equipped to do a cleanup, so you won't be sitting in anything unsavory for long.

After your baby's head has fully emerged, they will turn one last time to face your side and slip their shoulders out. And the rest of their body will follow.

Finally, the nine long months are OVER!

Oh, wait. Sorry. One last thing.

Stage 3

The afterbirth

Though it would be nice to leave the world behind to enjoy uninterrupted snuggles with your newborn, if you deliver vaginally, there is one final step before you are truly done with birth: delivering the placenta, or, as it's also known, the afterbirth.

The placenta, the magical organ that grew from scratch to nourish and take care of your baby during pregnancy, is no longer necessary. Usually, it comes out between five and thirty minutes following birth, and sometimes in the emotional rush of seeing your baby for the first time, you may not notice it's happening. You'll experience mild contractions (especially compared to what was going on earlier) that help move the placenta through the birth canal, and your midwife or doctor may apply pressure to your uterus or even tug lightly on the cord to speed things along. Sometimes they administer a shot of oxytocin, which helps minimize postpartum bleeding and to expel the placenta, and shrinks the uterus. Once the placenta is out, it will be examined, and if it is intact, you're back to bonding time with that freshly baked baby.

C-SECTIONS

Cesarean (no relation to Julius Caesar), or C-sections, a.k.a. belly births, are the most common major surgical procedure performed today. C-sections can be prescheduled due to medical conditions or obstetrical complications, like a breech baby, or in the case of multiples. They can also happen unexpectedly during vaginal deliveries if the cord becomes tangled, in cases of placental abruption or previa (when the placenta is covering part or all of the cervix), if labor stops progressing, and in cases of uterine rupture, a baby in distress, a baby too large for the pelvis, or when labor stalls out. For sufferers of sexual assault or abuse, C-sections can reduce associations with trauma. However, because they are so common, there is a perception that they pose fewer risks and involve less pain than delivering vaginally, leading some women to want to schedule them without a medical need.

The main reasons cited in the case of scheduled C-sections without a medical indication are convenience and control over the timing of birth, anxiety related to labor pain, and fear of urinary incontinence and stretching. While the idea of not laboring for hours or days is, let's be honest, appealing, if you're thinking about it for these reasons, there are considerations to weigh. Not to mention that your doctor may not perform C-sections on maternal request.

C-sections are major abdominal surgery. Your hospital stay will be two to four days—twice that of a vaginal birth—and at-home recovery is typically several weeks longer. Planned C-sections are associated with increased risk of postpartum complications and infection versus vaginal delivery and present a higher risk of maternal death and uterine rupture in future pregnancies. You will also be left with an abdominal scar, which is usually covered by your underwear or bathing suit but will take time to heal. Sometimes it's possible to do a trial of labor or vaginal birth after C-section (TOLAC or VBAC), depending what instigated the first one, but it's not always possible. If you're trying to avoid incontinence, studies have shown that it is just as likely to happen after a C-section as a vaginal birth (the pelvic floor stretches a lot during pregnancy), and that at best, the rate is just 8 percent lower.

Ultimately, the decision should be made after a discussion weighing the pros and cons with your physician, as there are many situations where a C-section is more beneficial than a vaginal birth. And if you do decide it's the best way, or if a medical reason pops up during a planned vaginal delivery, getting a C-section doesn't mean you will be any less of a parent or failed a test. The goal is a healthy baby and a healthy mom. C-sections are often necessary to make that happen.

How it starts is dependent on what led you to a C-section. If it was planned, the whole experience is pretty chill. If it's an emergency, it will be more intense. The whole surgery takes between forty-five minutes and one hour from start to finish.

The first step is receiving an epidural and IV that will numb your lower body and allow for the delivery of other medications. Next, you'll be moved to the operating room, where the doctors will set up the surgical field and clean your stomach. There will be a curtain draped between you and where they cut, though many hospitals now provide a "gentle C-section" option, which means the curtain is dropped so you can see your baby as they are lifted out.

Today's C-section incisions are discreet, and around four to six inches long. Most cuts are horizontal and happen below your bikini line (hence why they are also known as bikini cuts). The first cut opens your skin, the second cuts through your fascia, and the third goes into your uterus. The baby is then lifted out. If everything is okay, your partner can cut the umbilical cord and you can try breastfeeding or have skin-to-skin time. The placenta will be removed after the cord is cut, and the last step is to stitch you up. Afterward, you'll head to recovery and then to your postpartum room.

So what does it feel like? Answer: not much. Once the epidural or spinal block kicks in, the only sensations are pressure and tugging, as the ob-gyn pushes on your abdomen to help deliver your baby, and sometimes cold from the freezing OR and medications. Nausea is another common side effect and can happen during or after surgery.

WHAT HAPPENS RIGHT AFTER BIRTH

Sometimes called the "golden hour," those first sixty minutes are your first opportunity to bond, try out breastfeeding if that's your plan, and enjoy that new-baby smell. The first physical assessments of your baby can be done while they are resting on your chest, and all the weighing, measuring, bathing, and other medical procedures can wait until later unless there are complications for one or both of you.

Events for baby

Your baby just entered the world, and it's already time for their first exams. When and whether they receive some of them is up to you, and something you put into your birth preferences. But it's important to understand what to expect, and to address any areas of strong preference with your care team before they're in the middle of it post-birth.

Apgar test

The Apgar test is typically given one and five minutes after birth to see if your baby needs any extra care. Named for its inventor, Dr. Virginia Apgar, it grades babies in five areas:

- Appearance (skin color—from bluish to nice pink color)
- Pulse (heart rate—from zero to more than 100 beats/ minute)
- Grimace (reflex irritability—from no reaction when very gently pinched to a cough or cry)
- Activity (muscle tone—from limp to active)
- Respiration (breathing effort—from no cry to strong cry)

Each category is worth two points, for a maximum Apgar score of ten. Babies who score a seven or more are considered very healthy. Perfectly healthy babies can have low Apgar scores at the minute mark, but 98 percent of babies reach a score of seven after five minutes out of the womb.

Cord clamping and cutting

We talked about it in the birth preferences, but delayed cord clamping allows more blood to flow to your baby's body in the first minutes after birth. This means instead of immediately cutting the cord when your baby arrives, there will be a pause until it stops pulsing, assuming there are no complications during birth. It is not possible to wait to cut the cord if there is an emergency with you or your baby.

Heel-stick test

Before you and your new addition leave the hospital, a few drops of your baby's blood are collected from their heel, in a procedure appropriately known as the heel-stick test. It screens for heritable and genetic conditions. It's done early in life because many heritable conditions can be treated before they cause any serious health problems.

Each state's public health department mandates screens for different conditions after a hospital birth, so if you'd like specifics, visit babysfirsttest.org to see what is offered in your area. Tests vary due to costs and laws, frequency of specific disorders in certain states, availability of treatments for each condition, and funding sources. Typically, you'll receive the results from your pediatrician a few weeks later.

Eye drops, vitamin K shot, bathing, circumcision, hepatitis B vaccine

The birth preferences you put together should address all of this. But as a reminder, there is a standard course of care that all infants born in hospitals receive. When and whether they receive some of them is up to you, so address this in the early stages of labor so your care team knows your preferences ahead of time.

Eye drops and the vitamin K shot are typically administered an hour after birth. The first bath is optional and can be delayed until you go home. If you give birth in a hospital, circumcision (if requested) usually happens within forty-eight hours of birth. It can also happen a few weeks later if it's done for religious reasons.

Hearing test

Ninety-eight percent of all newborns receive this screening. Babies with hearing challenges require special care. Early interventions can improve their development, communication, and language abilities. It is quick and painless and can be done while they are sleeping.

There are two methods to screen newborn hearing. The first uses headphones to play tones and clicks, and electrodes on the baby's head measure their brain response. The second method measures the response when clicks are played into the baby's ears through a tiny probe in their ear canal.

Congenital heart defect screening

The critical congenital heart defect (CCHD) test looks for low oxygen levels, which can indicate issues with your baby's heart. This is another noninvasive, painless screening that happens twenty-four hours after birth. A small sensor will be attached to your baby's skin, then connected to an oximeter, which measures their oxygen levels. Around 7,200 babies per year are born with CCHDs, and may need surgery or help in the first year of life.

THE POSTPARTUM STAY

In the case of a C-section, once you're stitched up, you'll be wheeled into a recovery room, then into your postpartum room for a few nights of observation. After a vaginal birth, you may stay in the same room or move to the postpartum ward, and if needed, receive stitches to repair any tears in your vagina and/or perineum. Expect a two-to-three-night stay after a C-section, and twenty-four to forty-eight hours for an uncomplicated vaginal birth.

If you plan to breastfeed, your baby will room in with you, or be brought in from the nursery every few hours. Don't beat yourself up if things are not working immediately. We'll get into this in greater detail later, but your milk can take time to come in—especially after a C-section. If you need assistance with breastfeeding, that's not only okay, it's normal.

Now that you've read what the textbooks say about childbirth, you probably wonder how mine went. Even though I was an overprepared person who understood every possible birth scenario, mine was a prime example of things not going according to plan.

Based on the nonstop kicks in the ribs, I assumed our son would spring into the world on time, or early. But as we approached forty-one weeks, at which point I was giant and impatient, he was still comfortably nestled in my abdomen, hiccupping away.

Knowing what I did about due date accuracy, I chose to give him a few more days to emerge voluntarily as all my check-ins were clear of issues. The induction was scheduled for forty-one weeks, three days, so two days before, I went in for a final monitoring session. The medical team suggested a second membrane sweep to encourage some action. Later that night, I woke up thinking I had wet the bed. No rom-com-style public gush for me—my water broke all over my pregnancy pillow while I was sleeping.

As the day wore on without any real contractions, I saw my cozy plan for labor at home with Nick, our dog, and doulas slip away. So after one last light dinner, we loaded up our go bags and drove to the hospital.

There was no wait in triage; we went straight into a labor and delivery room, since my bag had already been open for eighteen hours, and I was technically past my due date. The first doctor urged an immediate Pitocin hookup to jump-start labor, but I demanded my full twenty-four hours (and a few critical hours of sleep) to see if things would start on their own. Thank goodness we did, because I needed rest for the adventure ahead.

Little guy still refused to budge, so at one to two centimeters dilated, I started on Pitocin early the next morning at the twenty-four-hour mark, with the dosage increasing every thirty minutes. After that, the contractions came on strong and suddenly, accompanied by intense nausea.

I chose not to get an epidural immediately, so I wasn't confined to bed. Instead, nitrous and the comfort measures we had practiced, like breathing, the TENS machine, and soaks in the tub, were my coping mechanisms. My memory of the ten hours I spent moving between the tub and bed and birthing stool and yoga ball is a complete blur. Though I tried my best to stay calm, eventually I coped by yelling into the nitrous mask at the peak of contractions (not recommended) and squeezing a small plastic comb in my hand like Dumbo and his magic feather as a distraction.

I've never been a modest person, and after all the pregnancy exams I didn't think I had any modesty left. But labor really put a nail in it. I started the day in my own cute hospital gown brought from home, but after my first trip to the tub, I was fully and un-

apologetically naked for the rest of it. Nudity isn't mandatory, of course, but if you're planning tub time during labor, it's probably how you'll end up.

Labor pain is hard to articulate. Friends described it as the worst menstrual cramps of their lives. My back felt alternately like an elephant was using it as a stool and my spine was ripping in half. Time in the tub helped, but it was still excruciating. I found out later that I was in back labor, as my son was stuck facing the wrong way.

A benefit of attempting vaginal birth with no epidural is that I could feel the little guy making the trip toward the exit. At times, I even felt an urge to bear down. However, early that evening, the movement ground to a halt. I noted the time and gave myself another hour to see if anything would change, but mentally prepared for another unexpected twist.

After discussing the options with Nick and our doula, and feeling zero progress after another hour, we decided it was time for an epidural to see if it would help me relax. However, I suspected his massive head was stuck, so I acknowledged to myself that a C-section might be required. If that happened, an epidural would be necessary anyway.

The decision was cemented after the most frustrating cervical exam of my life. After ten hours of intense labor and Pitocin, I was still only four centimeters dilated, and not fully effaced. The amniotic sac had been open for almost forty-eight hours, which meant infection was increasingly possible.

The astounding pain relief from the epidural melted those concerns away temporarily. I was bummed not to be able to get out of bed, but after such a long day, it was a welcome break. On went the hospital gown, up went the Pitocin, and in went the Foley catheter (a tube that goes into the bladder to drain urine), which oddly didn't work even after it was inserted a second time.

After a somewhat restful night, the Pitocin was maxed out, and I was still only five centimeters dilated. My cervix also had a lip that was impeding his progress. And there was more bad news. My white blood cell count was elevated, which meant chorio-amnionitis, an infection in my uterus. My creatinine levels were high, indicating my kidneys were no longer doing their job. And the catheter still wasn't working twelve hours later. The combination of symptoms led the team to conclude I had preeclampsia with severe features, which meant a magnesium sulfate drip to avoid progression to eclampsia, a sometimes-deadly condition.

Knowing the goal was a vaginal birth, the medical team gave us a few more hours before we had to talk plan B. When we hit the deadline, I was only at six centimeters dilated, my bag had been open for over sixty hours, and little dude's heart rate started to spike.

That's when I called it.

Watching the medical team mobilize for the C-section made me feel like a patient in a medical procedural. Within fifteen minutes I was wheeled into a brightly lit operating room, surrounded by what seemed like dozens of doctors, and lifted onto a skinny bed. The drape was raised, more pain management hit, Nick and our doula sat by my side, and the procedure began. Though I was alert, considering the volume of pharmaceuticals coursing through my body, my focus was less on whatever they were doing to me and more on our labor playlist, which we brought into the OR. Mixed with the whoosh that I later found out was compressed air to create space in my abdomen, the music was a perfect distraction from the light pressure I felt as they tried to fish our baby out.

Then, the sound every new parent dreams about: the first cry. His outraged scream marked the most incredible moment of my life. And even more surreal—he was no longer an abstract bump. He was a tiny human with lungs and vocal cords that Nick and I made.

The drape was dropped, and for the first time, I saw our beautiful little boy. And he had quite the cone head after so much time wedged in my pelvis. We later found out his head was stuck and crushing my ureter, hence why I hadn't peed in nearly eighteen hours. It also meant the preeclampsia diagnosis was incorrect.

After a quick check of his vitals, Nick cut the cord and they brought him over to me. The medications had stirred up some serious nausea, so it wasn't the perfect skin-to-skin session I'd envisioned. But the relief that he was out and healthy trumped any disappointment in how it ended.

In the anemic weeks recovering from the C-section, I thought about what we could have done differently and replayed the experience with Nick and our doulas. We all agreed we might skip the membrane sweeps, but probably would have ended up in the same spot (though I maintain that my vagina *is* HUGE!!!).

Failure to progress and overreaction to jumps on the fetal monitor are gray areas that warrant more research and could help reduce the rate of unnecessary C-sections. In our situation, given the liters of fluid locked up in my bladder with no escape path and spikes on my labs, I couldn't stick to vaginal birth at any cost.

I did every bit of research possible (hell, I wrote the sections on birth right before it happened) and planned for the experience that I wanted. And I'll admit it: I thought none of this would happen to me because I was so prepared. Did I want a vaginal birth? Yes. And I endured over sixty hours of labor, advocated for myself, and took every possible route to make that happen. In the days before C-sections, I probably would have died, as my pelvis just wasn't big enough to accommodate my baby's giant head.

Third-Trimester Checklist

- ☐ Attend birth class (look into breastfeeding and infant care and CPR too).
- ☐ Take a tour of your chosen hospital or center before birth.
- ☐ Talk to work about the final details of your maternity leave.
- ☐ Apply to add your baby to insurance (this can also be done after birth, depending on your policy).
- ☐ Choose a pediatrician.
- ☐ Read a book about the first months home with an infant (there is an overview next to get you started).
- ☐ Preregister for your hospital or birth center stay.
- ☐ Book your six-week (or sooner!) postpartum visit, which you can project using your due date.
- ☐ Pack your hospital bag (don't forget partner and baby!).
- ☐ Prep the nursery (wash clothes and blankets so everything is ready).
- ☐ Finalize post-birth support and back-to-work childcare.
- ☐ Take a few maternity photos (no professional required—your friend or partner can play photographer).
- ☐ Set aside time to take care of yourself (pedicure, yoga, face mask—whatever makes you feel pampered and good).
- ☐ Plan post-birth meals (freeze meals and let friends and family help).
- ☐ Schedule a last pre-baby date night with your partner.
- ☐ Install your car seat (can't leave the hospital without it!).
- ☐ Stock up on postpartum items.

The Fourth Trimester

It's all over! You're no longer pregnant and have a brand-new baby in your arms. Mission: Accomplished. Right?

Wrong!

Back in the days of living in villages and multigenerational households, there was more exposure to pregnancy and its aftermath. But in today's nuclear families, much of our collective perspective comes from polished narratives on social media. So in the spirit of continued honesty and not avoiding the hard parts, here is a sneak peek into what life is like in the fourth trimester.

Your body will be a constipated, deflated, leaking hot mess of hormones, oddly colored discharge, and milk in those first weeks after birth. You will be sleep-deprived. Your mind will be fuzzy. The hormonal surges won't stop even though the baby exited your body. And the mental transition from pregnant to parent is huge. Most new parents, if they're candid, will admit that they had to throw their expectations out the window and just go with the flow.

Some parents immediately feel a swell of indescribable love for their baby at birth. But if it takes a while for you to bond, there's nothing wrong. Infants emerge helpless, without the ability to clearly communicate their needs, and there is a lot of guesswork before you figure them out. You'd think the nine months of bodily cohabitation mean you already know each other well, but every baby has a set of opinions, preferences, and personality all their own. And your ability to mold and shape this tiny human will be limited by who they are when they pop out.

During your stay in the postpartum wing, you'll be surrounded by nurses, lactation consultants, pediatricians, and ob-gyns who will check in, help swaddle or put the baby to sleep, and dispense as much or as little advice as you'd like. Then at some point, you and your partner will find yourselves standing outside the hospital with your brand-new baby snug in a car seat, thinking, *Now what?*

If you thought there were strong opinions about how to manage your pregnancy "the right way," just wait for the pressure related to breastfeeding, shedding pregnancy weight, and managing baby-related accessories and routines when you get home. The mom-on-mom judgment is ruthless, and is the hardest criticism to handle, since it's so unexpected.

Knowing all of this, be open to help. Remember what the word *partner* means and find ways to let yours pitch in, whether it's just holding the baby for a while, doing some feedings, taking over chores, dealing with diapers, or keeping you company while you're trapped on the couch resting and breastfeeding. For friends and family who offer general assistance, let them provide meals or do tasks like laundry. Prefer not to have visitors? There are delivery services that can reduce your long list of to-dos.

Most of this section is about you and your recovery. However, since baby isn't a native language for new parents and they don't arrive with a manual, we'll also explore their basic behaviors to help you decipher—and hopefully reduce—the tears. For all of you.

POSTPARTUM WARNING SIGNS

On a more serious note, the postpartum period is full of well-established issues, but health risks do not end at birth. If something doesn't feel right, you know your body and mind best, so share your symptoms with your partner and contact your care team.

Call your provider	• Blood pressure at or exceeding 140/90 (consider buying and keeping a cuff at home to self-monitor for the first ten days) • Severe headache that doesn't improve with medication • Swelling, redness, or pain in your hands, calves, thighs, or face • Vision changes • Stomach pain or nausea and vomiting • Chills or fever • Heart palpitations • Redness or severe pain in breasts • If your pain increases over time or requires more medication • Bright red bleeding that saturates more than two pads in an hour or if there are clots larger than an egg • Difficulty or pain urinating, or frequent urination with only small amounts each time • Thoughts of hurting yourself or your baby
Go to the ER or dial 911	• Blood pressure over 160/110 • Shortness of breath or trouble breathing • Seeing spots • Seizures

Mr. Baby (a nickname my son earned for looking like a full-grown man straight out of the womb, and for his adult-volume burps) was plunked into my arms in the recovery room.

Hours later, knowing movement helps with recovery, I was out of bed. By day two, I could slowly shuffle around the ward with Nick, who was pushing Mr. Baby in his wheeled crib.

To have the privilege of catheter removal, you must pee on your own, or it goes right back in. My plumbing was off, courtesy of Mr. Baby's head crushing my ureter, so it took a few tries before I was disconnected. In the meantime, I carried the bag of urine around like a little pet. It was not, however, a convenient accessory when I was ready for a shower. Between that, an IV hookup, and a chair to lean on, it was both the most logistics-heavy shower I've ever taken (where does one hang a bag of urine in a hospital shower?) and also, the GOAT. For me, there was nothing more life-affirming than rinsing it all off.

The "Now what?" moment didn't hit until we arrived home. We thought we had everything we needed for those early days, but, as with birth, there were many things we didn't anticipate. Like Mr. Baby's Houdini-like ability to escape from every swaddle type but one. How many wipes we would blow through cleaning off poop that had traveled up his back. Or that he was too long for newborn clothes after a few days and needed toddler-size socks for his hobbit feet.

Even with amazing support and visitors around to pitch in, the first weeks home were a blur. My brain was different, my body was different, and life in general was unrecognizable. Not to mention we had a tiny, bellowing stranger around whose needs we didn't fully (or at all) understand.

Navigating stairs and getting in and out of bed were very uncomfortable. As during pregnancy, getting up with a C-section incision required a roll to the side, versus sitting up straight. That mistake was painful enough that I only made it once. My legs looked inflated, thanks to the many medications I received during birth. Compression leggings helped until the fluid and swelling disappeared.

The only medications I took after my C-section were Tylenol and Motrin, on a rotating three-hour schedule. The combo was effective, unless I got behind the pain. Managing the timing for the different pills on top of infant feedings was impossible until I set recurring reminders on my phone. Odd hours was Motrin, even was Tylenol.

And then there were the night sweats. My God. The drenching night sweats lasted for two weeks. It felt like waking up in a sauna. I kept a towel next to the bed or put one under me as I slept, or the sheets would be soaked. Triggered by the fear that the effort would rip my sutures, I was hopelessly constipated. It took a combo of a laxative, a stool softener, and, finally, a suppository for me to get things moving. Trips to the bathroom were not productive (or too productive) for weeks. And rather than disappearing after pregnancy, my acid reflux intensified, making it hard to swallow.

In case you were wondering whether weighing yourself in the first six weeks is a good idea, I did so you don't have to. The first day home, my weight was the same as the day I left for the hospital. Seventy-two hours of horrific night sweats later, it dropped twenty pounds. That's right—TWENTY POUNDS OF FLUID RETENTION LOST IN THREE DAYS. Seriously, postpartum weight fluctuations make no sense. Give your body time to recover, stop worrying that you'll never fit into your prepregnancy jeans, and STEP AWAY FROM THE SCALE.

SO WHAT'S HAPPENING OUT THERE?

Month 1

Baby: Newborns have no sense of day and night and no idea that their arms and legs are attached to their body, since they do not yet understand what a body is! Their first days and weeks will mostly consist of sleeping, eating, snuggling, soiling diapers, and crying. They can't see much or very far, and their lack of muscle makes them feel fragile and floppy. Their eyes sometimes cross (when they're open), and there may be hiccups. But, man, do they smell good. Soak it in, as that delicious newborn fragrance doesn't last forever.

You: The first month after birth is pretty wild. Your breasts fill with milk, your hormones and emotions ricochet up and down, and your former bump shrinks. The swelling and fluid retention vanish mostly in the form of sweating and peeing. Postpartum bleeding, known as lochia, will also include other random discharge, and lasts in some form for six to eight weeks. You might experience a touch (or a lot) of incontinence, as everything is stretched after pregnancy and birth. The baby blues or more serious depression can kick in, too, so if you are experiencing any downs, talk to someone you trust. Walking is the safest and best activity you can do—regardless of how great you may feel—in the first six weeks.

Month 2

Baby: At the four- to six-week mark, your baby will be less lump-like and begin to do things like whip out a heart-melting smile. Cooing and gurgling can also start around now. The primary activities are still sleeping, eating, soiling diapers, and crying, though your baby will start to stay awake longer and be more interactive. It's a good time to introduce more visual stimuli (they love high-contrast, black-and-white images), or to test their grip using a rattle or other baby-safe toy. But warning: If they avoid eye contact or flap their arms wildly, you're in the overstimulation zone, and it's time for quiet.

You: Everyone's recovery after birth is different, and much of it depends on how your baby is eating and sleeping, and whether you are getting any rest. Bleeding should diminish, and if you aren't breastfeeding, the lochia may be replaced by your period. Yes, it can come back that fast. Ovulation can occur in the weeks even before your period returns, so if you are having sex, use some form of birth control (unless you'd like to care for two children under the age of one). It's also time to get your pelvic floor back in shape, especially if you are experiencing any leaks or laxity. Your postpartum checkup happens this month, so plan to chat about any issues, physical or mental (and get birth control recommendations). One in five women reports depression during the first three months postpartum (and this number is assumed to be low), so if this is you, seek the care you need.

Month 3

Baby: Sleep is still the primary activity, but the time between naps will continue to increase, which means more time for play. The daily routine may take on a more consistent pattern, and goes something like: Wake, change diaper, feed, burp, play, change diaper, sleep, repeat. Every baby has a different internal clock, and everyone's parenting preferences are different. Hands are the star attraction this month, and those tiny fists will be in your baby's mouth a lot. If you stick your baby in front of a mirror, they may not know it's their own reflection staring back, but it's entertaining to see them try to figure it out.

You: Postpartum hair loss can start around now, which means you may find larger-than-usual clumps of hair in your brush and shower. If your baby is sleeping for longer spans you may start to feel more rested; otherwise, the cumulative effects of sleep deprivation can be intense. Monitor your mental health, and make sure you have enough support. For many working moms, this is the last month at home. With that in mind, if you are breastfeeding and haven't begun pumping, you'll need to start, and introduce a bottle well in advance of your return to work.

Fourth-trimester symptoms and solutions

Uterine contractions

- When does it happen?
  Mostly in the two to three days right after birth, especially while breastfeeding

- Symptoms
  Uncomfortable cramping and bleeding. It can be intense and feel like labor contractions.

- Cause
  Your uterus has to shrink from its watermelon size at birth back down to a fist, a process called involution. Breastfeeding stimulates the release of oxytocin, which in turn causes contractions. Your uterus will be back to its original size six weeks after birth, though this process can take longer with subsequent pregnancies.

- Solutions
  Wait it out, unfortunately. Naproxen or ibuprofen are the most common medication recommendations, as they are allowed while

breastfeeding. Acetaminophen and aspirin come with side effects. A TENS machine can help you manage this pain.

The baby blues

- When does it happen?
  May have started during pregnancy, but can kick into gear any-time after birth, most commonly in the first two weeks

- Symptoms
  Loss of interest in activities you used to love; decreased ability to feel pleasure; feelings of worthlessness, fear, or guilt, or suicidal thoughts

- Cause
  Hormonal swings, physical shifts in your body, major life changes

- Solutions
  Speak to your partner or someone else you trust, schedule an ap-pointment with your doctor, contact a mental health professional, join a mom support group, or schedule a virtual appointment.

Excessive sweating, especially as night sweats

- When does it happen?
  For the first weeks postpartum; peaks at two weeks, then tapers off

- Symptoms
  Waking up feeling like you just walked out of a steam room or shower, regardless of the temperature

- Cause

Your body's way of getting rid of the fluids you accumulated during pregnancy or from medications given during birth. It's also triggered by low estrogen levels.

- Solutions

Sleep on a towel (or keep one at the ready), drink more fluids, take a cool bath and go to bed with wet hair, and make sure your bedroom is a cool temperature.

Hair loss

- When does it happen?

Around three months postpartum. Will return to normal six to twelve months after birth, based on where you are in the growth cycle.

- Symptoms

Finding more hair than usual in your shower and brush, sometimes in clumps

- Cause

Pregnancy and prenatal vitamins prevent hair from falling out at its normal rate. As soon as you give birth and your hormones drop, so too will your lush extra hairs.

- Solutions

Change up your shampoo and conditioner, try a different style or cut, use a volumizer, and keep taking that prenatal vitamin, especially if you are breastfeeding.

Fatigue

- **When does it happen?**
  Forever?

- **Symptoms**
  Inability to keep your eyes open or form coherent sentences, generally feeling drained at all times

- **Cause**
  You gave birth and are now taking care of a newborn. Breastfeeding can also contribute, as it takes even more energy to produce milk.

- **Solutions**
  Ask for help, go for a walk (seems counterintuitive, but it works!), employ all cheat codes such as food delivery and helpful friends, hydrate, sleep when the baby sleeps (even if just for a few minutes at a time).

Bleeding

- **When does it happen?**
  Heaviest in the first ten days after birth, it can last for four to six weeks. It also intensifies during and after breastfeeding as your uterus contracts.

- **Symptoms**
  Period-like bleeding that goes from red and pink to brown, and eventually yellow. If you see large clots, you fill a pad every hour, or there is a strong odor, call your provider.

- Cause

  Known as lochia, it's your body's way of getting rid of the extra blood, uterine tissue, and mucus left over from pregnancy.

- Solutions

  No tampons allowed for six weeks after birth (whether it was vaginal or C-section), so once you run out of the hospital's mesh panties, it's pads for heavy days and period underwear or liners as things subside. Too much physical activity too soon will trigger increased bleeding, so take it easy. And opt for dark pants until it stops.

Perineal discomfort

- When does it happen?

  The exact time frame varies widely, but it is typically weeks or months after birth.

- Symptoms

  Varying degrees of specific pain if you had stitches, general discomfort, and numbness, made worse by coughing, sneezing, or laughing

- Cause

  The stretching and pushing during birth, and the pressure of carrying a baby around for nine months. This pain isn't limited to vaginal births—you can also expect to have some discomfort with a C-section, especially if you labored first.

- Solutions

  Start your pelvic floor exercises, sit on a donut (not the kind with sugar), pour or squirt water on the area with a peri bottle, use padsicles (recipe to follow), take a sitz bath, apply numbing agents, wear loose bottoms.

Incontinence (urine or poop)

- When does it happen?

  Can start during pregnancy, and goes days, weeks, months, or even years postpartum if not treated

- Symptoms

  Leaking urine, poop, or poop juice while laughing, sneezing, jumping, lifting, and running. Can also manifest as a sudden urge to pee outside of normal bathroom activities.

- Cause

  Like perineal discomfort, it's caused by the pressure the baby put on your pelvic floor during pregnancy, and stretching during birth.

- Solutions

  Strengthening your pelvic floor with at-home exercises or seeing a pelvic floor therapist is step one. If you are experiencing fecal incontinence, have your anal tone checked by your ob-gyn.

Trouble pooping

- When does it happen?

  May be a sequel to pregnancy constipation, but can also start directly after birth and most commonly lasts for the first two weeks

- Symptoms

  Manifests as constipation and pain every time you try to go to the bathroom, or as the opposite problem—diarrhea and loose stool

- Cause

Post-birth pain medications and iron supplements make this worse, as can a sore perineum (the first poop after birth is kind of terrifying).

- Solutions

Eat fiber-packed foods (grains, fruit, legumes), drink plenty of fluids (you'll need it to make breast milk), take a walk. And if your provider offers stool softeners, say "Yes, please."

Hemorrhoids

- When does it happen?

Might have started during pregnancy, and can last for months postpartum

- Symptoms

Pain when you sit or go to the bathroom, itching, and bleeding

- Cause

Swollen veins in your anus and lower rectum, caused by straining during pregnancy, birth, or trips to the bathroom

- Solutions

Eat a high-fiber diet, spot treat with witch hazel or Tucks pads, stay hydrated, and try stool softeners.

Nipple Pain

- When does it happen?

Felt mostly during breastfeeding or while pumping

- Symptoms
Tenderness or bleeding and cracking nipples, usually made worse during breastfeeding

- Cause
A bad latch or bad positioning while breastfeeding, or vigorous sucking

- Solutions
Work on the underlying problem to avoid making it worse. Nipple butter and creams can help, along with cold compresses. Talk to a lactation consultant if it persists.

Blocked ducts or mastitis

- When does it happen?
Any time while breastfeeding or pumping

- Symptoms
Pain in breast tissue or a lump in the breast that is tender to the touch

- Cause
Can happen when a bra doesn't fit or is too tight, after engorgement, or if a nipple or duct is blocked

- Solutions
Massage your breast in the shower or use a warm compress before feedings. If you experience body aches and a fever over 100.4 degrees Fahrenheit along with the other symptoms, you may have an infection called mastitis, and should call your doctor immediately. You can get sepsis from untreated mastitis, so please take it seriously.

FOR PARTNERS

You watched your significant other go through pregnancy and child-birth (miraculous what the human body is capable of, right?), and now your job is to help her recover while transitioning to your own new identity as a parent. Don't forget about that communication practice you did during pregnancy. More than ever, it's important to check in and keep an eye out for any signs she is struggling or has health symptoms that indicate something serious is going on. Share responsibilities related to the baby and give her space and time to take care of herself (and catch up on sleep!).

There is a tremendous amount of pressure—external and self-imposed—on women to be perfect mothers and partners, while also performing at work and bouncing back physically. Don't wait for her to ask for help—ask what she needs. Be proactive and offer up whatever assistance you can, as often as you can, and own the tasks you take on.

Around 10 percent of all new dads experience paternal postpar-tum depression (and this estimate is suspected to be low), so don't be surprised if you feel yourself struggling emotionally too. Changes in household roles, financial concerns, new responsibilities, feelings about intimacy and sex, and return-to-work issues can all contribute. Women receive a standardized screening for postnatal depression. Men, not so much. Though the research is scant, we suspect half of men whose partners experience PPD will struggle with it too.

Men are now taking more equal parenting roles and want to be involved dads. But they do not always open up to friends and fam-ily when they experience mental or physical health challenges. Men experience more loneliness during fatherhood, with less than half of men report feeling satisfied with their friendships, and in one survey, only one in five said they received emotional support from a friend in the preceding week. While there are many groups and communities for moms, dads have decidedly fewer options—online and in person. Suffering alone can lead to feelings of resentment toward your child or partner and ruin the early days as a new parent or have far more serious consequences. If you need help, please don't ignore how you're feeling and speak to a medical provider.

Be her healthcare champion

During pregnancy, the focus is all on mom. After birth, that attention shifts to the baby. Your most important job is keeping both mom and baby safe, and that means ensuring that her health is not sidelined. Postpartum preeclampsia is increasingly common (30 percent of all preeclampsia presents postpartum), and the simplest way to detect it is through blood pressure, hence why you're reading again how important it is to have a cuff around. Blood pressure goes up with lack of sleep (make sure she is napping), so check it daily to see if it hits the levels indicated in the chart earlier (140/90 means a call to her provider, 160/110 or above means an immediate trip to the ER or call 911). If she starts bleeding more or the discharge turns from darker red back to bright red days or weeks after birth, that can mean she's been doing too much—make her rest.

Role-playing

This has a different meaning in a post-baby world (though, if done well and often, is a massive turn-on—not that your partner is ready for sex right now!). You may already have a solid division of labor, and if so, you're ahead of most couples. If you don't, here are a few places to start:

- **Chief sanitation officer:** You change the diaper, she breastfeeds, you burp your new addition before he goes back to sleep.
- **Top chef:** Not a great cook? Now is a great time to learn easy recipes, the art of ordering in, or to say yes to that meal train from friends and family.
- **Vice president of errand running:** Gearing up a baby to go to the store can take longer than the trip itself.

Offer to do errands, or, if she wants to get out of the house, to spend some time with the little one while she is gone.

- **Head of people:** The first weeks home are packed with eager family and friends who want to meet the baby. It can be a lot to manage as a new mom, especially if people overstay their welcome. Set a schedule and expectations around visit duration (and any specific preferences around handling the baby) so she doesn't have to.

Create some me-time (for her)

This may be something as simple as a hot bath or going for a walk alone or with a friend. She may not ask for it, and she may even turn you down the first few times you suggest it (mom guilt is real), but keep offering, and encourage her to do it. The benefit for you is solo bonding time with your baby—important, as you should be able to take over for your partner in the event of an emergency. These early sessions can have a lasting and positive impact on your long-term relationship with your baby, too.

Help with breastfeeding and night feedings

Taking over one of the night feedings is perhaps the kindest way to help your partner start feeling like more of a human and less like a deflated zombie. Even if you can't do it in the first few weeks because she's exclusively breastfeeding, offer your company and help. Hanging out with a thirsty baby is tiring, repetitive, and, at times, lonely work. Bring her snacks or drinks, help her get more comfortable, wash bottles and pump parts, burp the baby, or just keep her entertained.

Become an early-parenting expert

During pregnancy, putting knowledge into practice was more about being empathetic and emotionally supportive for your partner. But now that your baby is here, you can take an equal role in the process of helping them learn and explore. Get to know the different stages of development and build an environment to help their curious mind grow. And when one phase has passed, pack up the toys (and clothes they've outgrown!) for a friend or future child.

Be patient in the bedroom

Sex after childbirth can take some time. The guideline is to wait six weeks after giving birth to let things down there heal, but if your partner experienced any trauma or tearing, it could be longer. In some cases, much longer. Her body isn't the same, and she may feel self-conscious about that, too. The first time is a little scary even if she's feeling okay, so talk about it first, and be gentle. Vaginal dryness is common, especially if she is breastfeeding, so if you get things going, keep lube at the ready.

Own specific tasks

A gripe cited by all moms (even those with amazing, involved partners) is the gender inequality of childcare and housework, which most research shows is two-thirds on the shoulders of women. It starts before kids and expands after they arrive, lasting all the way through childhood. There are many approaches to making things more equitable, but the most basic rule is to assign and take full ownership over specific tasks versus splitting things up, asking ad hoc constantly, keeping score, and expecting each other to be a mind reader and "know" what to do. This means divvying up key tasks that each of you can 100 percent own (while again, not keeping score). These can be anything from taking out the trash or doing laundry to managing childcare or drops-offs and other baby-related activities. The key is to build trust in each other, so when a task is assigned, the other person doesn't have to worry about it getting done.

RECOVERY

Managing your body, mental health, nutrition, and birth control postpartum

In China, some new moms practice *zuo yue zi*, or "sitting in," the month after birth. They stay at home and rest while a live-in assistant cooks and handles childcare. South Korea takes this idea of sitting in a step further with *joriwon*, an all-inclusive resort for postnatal care. For two weeks, mothers' bodies are pampered and all meals are provided, along with massages, yoga, laundry, and housekeeping. The Netherlands has a service called *kraamzorg* that sends a maternity nurse over every day for up to two weeks after birth. The nurse checks in on you and the baby, answers questions, and also does household chores and runs to the grocery store. The service is reimbursed almost entirely by basic health insurance policies.

You get the idea—support systems exist because recovery after birth takes time and help. Care in the US is not quite so focused on a mom's well-being, and there is no luxurious spa-like environment waiting to welcome you and your newborn—unless you can pay for it out of pocket.

While a trip to the pediatrician will happen a few days after you go home, the first appointment to check on you may not be for six weeks. Making contact with your care team in the first three weeks is encouraged, but it is not a standard of care yet. A bonus of working with a doula is that they typically do a home visit shortly after birth to check in and help with recovery, breastfeeding, and general well-being. And there are postpartum doulas who can provide extra help, especially if you do not have family around, are a single mom, or have a partner who must go back to work. Other than that, unless you utilize telemedicine, tap into your broader network of providers, or have someone else to help, you're on your own.

Only 60 percent of women attend their six-week postpartum checkup. Letting it slide makes sense deep in newborn land. You're tired, and it's easier to put aside your own needs than your baby's. But your health is important, too—as a caretaker, food source, and giver of love and affection. The low attendance rate is why the pediatrician will ask how you are doing and if you have enough help. Pediatricians are the first line of defense in identifying postpartum depression and other problems with parents, so be honest.

When—not if! (take the baby; your provider will love meeting them!)—you attend your postpartum appointment, discussion topics will range from how you are doing physically and checking your incision if you had a C-section or perineal recovery from a vaginal birth, to pregnancy spacing (how long you plan to wait if you're having another child) and birth control, feeding your baby, medical conditions you are managing, and emotional wellness. If you're given the all-clear, you'll see your ob-gyn again a year later for a normal appointment.

SCREW GETTING YOUR OLD BODY BACK

Your social media feeds are filled with toned abs and perky boobs on infant-toting women wearing bikinis mere weeks after giving birth. So it must be easy to get that body you miss back, right?

Yeah, no. Mommy tucks, Photoshop, personal trainers, good lighting, and strategic angles all make it look a lot easier than it is. And there's another secret. That old body you had before pregnancy? It's gone. Poof. Sorry. Your body will never be exactly the same again. Instead of pining for the original version, it's time to celebrate body 2.0. Yes, it's a little more stretched, and if you decide to step on a scale (please don't for a while!), the number you'll see will probably be higher than you'd like. But this new body pulled off GROWING AND BIRTHING A HUMAN BEING. So be proud and cut that amazing body some freaking slack.

Your uterus will shrink from watermelon size back to a closed fist just six weeks after birth, which will flatten out your bump considerably. The most noticeable contraction happens in the first three days, especially during and after breastfeeding. Your abs will begin to knit back together as your uterus contracts, but it takes eight weeks or longer for them to close the gap entirely. Your pelvic floor can take up to a year to recover, as it was stretched to three times its normal limit during pregnancy and birth. If you're breastfeeding, you will hold on to a bit of extra fat until the baby weans. Your thyroid, a.k.a. the controller of your metabolism, can experience changes that make it harder for you to lose weight after pregnancy, too.

Body dysmorphia is common during and after pregnancy and can be serious. It can manifest as fear, feelings of lost control, or in conditions like pregorexia, which is anorexia in pregnant and postpartum women. Having trouble relating to physical changes is normal, but if you are unable to let things go, talk to someone and cut your social media consumption, especially if it's causing you to obsess.

WALK BEFORE YOU RUN

If you're an active person and worked out during pregnancy, the six-week exercise break right after birth can be difficult, especially if you are itchy to get back to it or feel pressure to shed baby weight. Why six weeks? It is the commonly accepted guideline for most injuries, and, after birth, enough time for the average body to heal. So, what can or should you do physically? The answer varies based on what happened during birth, how you gave birth, and how you're healing. Unless you are on bed rest, the single best exercise for your pelvic floor, physical recovery, and sanity after six weeks is walking. Walks with the stroller are invigorating (given it's not Minnesota in January), and a great way to soothe a fussy newborn and give you a break from cabin fever, too.

To avoid issues like prolapse or diastasis, stick to gentle movement for the first six weeks, and don't lift anything heavy other than the baby (challenging if you already have another child at home!). Going too hard too fast can set back your recovery, so take it slow. Trust your body—pain is its way of telling you to stop and pay attention. Once your baby's neck is stable, you can add them to your workouts, and there are plenty of mom-and-me classes to explore.

Moves for the first six weeks

Light stretching for a few minutes while your baby is hanging out next to you is a great way to regain flexibility and move your body, especially if you're experiencing the mom lean or the breastfeeding hunch. If you loved cat/cow during pregnancy, add the following two stretches and make it a daily five-minute routine.

Chest opener

Household items like a scarf, a long resistance band, a belt, or even a mop or broom handle are all you need for this one.

- While standing, hold your item of choice at tension in front of your body.
- Keep your arms straight and bring the item over your head as far as you can.
- Stop if you feel any shoulder pain.

Figure four

This deep stretch is the ultimate release.

- Lie on your back and cross your ankle over your knee.
- Using your hands, bring the four shape into your chest.
- Hold for a few breaths, then release and repeat on the other side.

After six weeks

Every person's body recovers differently, and your rate of progress is dependent on what happened during birth and any body trauma from pregnancy. Once you clear your six-weeks postpartum appointment, there are a few more movements to add to your routine, and you can start to explore the activities you did before pregnancy. Postpartum recovery doesn't happen overnight, and for the best long-term results, ease into it. You can bring back glute kickbacks and add these two moves to find stability in your body.

Bridges

A quick and easy way to regain stability in your core and back while you stretch

- Lie on your back with your knees bent and your knees and feet hip-width apart.
- Press your pelvis up toward the ceiling and squeeze your butt.
- Lower back down to the floor one vertebra at a time, starting at the top and ending at your tailbone.
- Try working up to ten reps, three times in a row.

Squats

Move slowly with control, as your postpartum
alignment may be a little off

- Use a chair as a prop until you are comfortable doing air squats. It's there to ensure your weight doesn't rock into the backrest.
- Slowly stand up and sit down for ten reps, three times in a row.
- As you squat, imagine there is an invisible straight line running along your head, shoulders, and tailbone—make sure you do not arch your back.

COMPLICATIONS

Hearing that your body and vagina stretch *a lot* during pregnancy and birth is no surprise. But there are three conditions that top the list of dirty, dirty postpartum secrets no one tells you. Perineal and vaginal tearing, diastasis recti, and pelvic organ prolapse affect millions of women to varying degrees, yet awareness of these conditions is very low.

France's *la rééducation périnéale*, a.k.a. a pelvic floor rehabilitation program designed to help manage these issues, is a standard of care for all women who give birth. Though there is no similar support in the US, consider channeling your inner French girl and making an appointment with a pelvic floor therapist. Unless they are out of network or don't accept it, insurance should cover these appointments. It's also important to get back into your Kegels and pelvic floor strengthening as soon as you can after giving birth. Even though you probably won't be able to feel them working for a while, trust that they are!

Dealing with diastasis

No matter how diligent you are, that stubborn post-pregnancy pooch can hang around for months and sometimes years after birth. Diastasis recti happens when the tissue in your abdominal muscles weakens and stretches during pregnancy to accommodate your growing baby. More than 60 percent of pregnant women experience diastasis in some degree, and it's not completely preventable.

The effects are not just cosmetic. A diastasis diagnosis can mean worse posture, lower-back pain, pelvic prolapse, increased risk of hernia, and more frequent instances of incontinence. Ugh. Your provider may check for it at your six-week appointment by measuring the width between your lower abs with their fingers. A one- or two-finger-width split is normal and will heal on its own. If it's wider, you may need to do some work to bring your abs back together.

The most successful way to treat diastasis is to target and strengthen your transverse abdominis (TVA), not go hard at the gym. Think of the TVA as your body's corset. It is the deep abdominal muscle that wraps around your torso. You'll learn more about this muscle if you work with a pelvic floor PT, and postpartum Pilates is another excellent way to work on your TVA and wake up your lower abdominals. If you're ready to fire up your TVA, here is a move to get you started.

Spinal compressions

- Lie on your back with your knees bent and your knees and feet hip-width apart.
- Press your spine into the floor as if you're smashing a bug with your lower back.
- Hold this abdominal contraction for three to four breaths, breathing in your upper ribs.
- Relax and release your abs.
- Repeat eight to ten times.

Just as important as rehabbing your TVA and pelvic floor is avoiding movements that make diastasis worse. Traditional ab exercises (sit-ups, crunches, roll-ups, curls), backbends, spinal extensions, and planks are some of the worst offenders. Avoid heavy lifting for the first six to eight weeks, and eat a fiber-rich diet to prevent constipation or straining.

Postpartum belly binding and wrapping is a tradition in many cultures, and there is evidence that especially during C-section recovery, it improves walking, controls pain, and helps overall with patient satisfaction. Let's be clear: This binder isn't designed to give you a snatched waist. We are talking about a medical-grade, elasticized, nothing-sexy-about-it binder designed specifically for the postpartum period. You may be offered one at the hospital—if you aren't, ask for one (or two—they get stretched in the first two weeks). There is some research that shows it can help your abs zip back together, but what you'll hear anecdotally from other moms is that binders make you feel more solid and held in while your organs are still all over the place.

I did not experience any diastasis, which I attribute in part to my careful avoidance of lifting heavy things and crunching motions. Also luck, genetics, and knowing about it beforehand. Eight weeks postpartum, I still did the roly-poly sit-up so I didn't put unwelcome pressure on my abs. I used an abdominal binder after both C-sections, starting in the hospital and for most of the first few weeks. While I can't attribute my relatively easy recoveries to it directly, I did love the way I felt pulled back together, and my abs did flatten out more quickly than I expected. My rib cage did not get that memo and took two years and intense Pilates after my second son arrived to contract back (mostly) to its prepregnancy state.

Perineal pain and tearing

Nearly all first-time mothers with vaginal births experience some amount of perineal pain and tearing. Sometimes, it means you will leave the hospital with a few stitches. Depending on the severity, activities like using the restroom, laughing, sneezing, and coughing will be painful for a few weeks, and you will experience some incontinence.

There are four classifications of tearing, and first- and second-degree tears are by far the most common. Around 4 percent of all tears are third- or fourth-degree, so when you read about them, don't panic.

- **First-degree:** minor tears of the vagina's mucosal tissue that don't generally require stitches
- **Second-degree:** vaginal tearing plus some perineal tearing that requires stitches
- **Third-degree:** vaginal tearing plus perineal tearing plus anal sphincter tearing that requires stitches and sometimes surgery
- **Fourth-degree:** tear all the way from vagina and perineum to anus requiring stitches and surgery

Though there are now healing foams and liners, bidets, and squirt bottles for a sore perineum, one classic solution is the padsicle. It is exactly what you'd guess—a menstrual pad that you soak in a brew of different healing agents, freeze, and put into your mesh underwear for cooling relief.

Padsicle recipe

Ingredients

4 tablespoons witch hazel (alcohol-free)
2 tablespoons aloe vera gel
1 to 2 drops of lavender essential oil
Your favorite thick menstrual pads
Spray bottle
Freezer bags
Freezer

Mix the witch hazel, aloe, and lavender oil and pour into a spray bottle. Pull out your menstrual pad of choice and spray on a layer of this concoction until it's wet but not soaked. Put the pad in a freezer bag and place it in the freezer. When it chills, ice down your perineum.

If you're not into frozen pads, the best ways to support recovery are to keep things clean and not mess with your stitches, squirt warm water while and after going to the bathroom (bidets are great for this if you want to upgrade your toilet), avoid constipation, sit on a donut pillow, and use a warm compress or take a sitz bath.

Pelvic organ prolapse

Women often describe pelvic organ prolapse (POP, the worst possible acronym for this condition) as their vagina falling out or the feeling of sitting on a ball. It happens when the bladder, uterus, small intestine, or rectum pushes against the vaginal wall, causing the vaginal wall to bulge outside of the vagina. It occurs most commonly after vaginal childbirth when the pelvic floor ligaments and fascia are stretched and can no longer hold the wall of the vagina up. POP can cause major issues like difficulty urinating and persistent back pain, and impacts the ability to exercise, especially running and jumping. Many sufferers avoid sex or intimacy due to the threat of incontinence.

POP is not a new condition. It is referenced in the Bible and in Egyptian hieroglyphics, with proposed treatments ranging from scaring things back into place with a hot poker, to tying a woman to a ladder upside down and shaking it. Thankfully, fumigating your vagina with herbs or dangling from a rope has been replaced by (you guessed it) pelvic floor PT and, when needed, surgery. More than two hundred thousand surgeries are performed each year to treat prolapse, and the number is climbing, so much so that there is a medical subspecialty called female pelvic medicine and reconstructive surgery (FPMRS) within urogynecology.

More than one in five women (that we know about—it's often not reported) experience POP, and the older you are, the more likely it is to happen. It is especially common when women hit menopause due to the drop in estrogen. It is difficult to diagnose because it may not be obvious in exams, or even a part of routine postpartum checkups. If you feel a lot of discomfort or experience continued incontinence or a backache that won't go away, you should talk to your provider. They'll prescribe PT or a pessary, which is a circular device inserted into the vagina to support the pelvic organs, before surgery is considered. If you're planning to have more children, many physicians will wait to perform surgery until you are all finished with pregnancy.

MANAGING YOUR MENTAL HEALTH

Right after birth, especially around day four, estrogen and progesterone drop. This can lead to anxiety and the "baby blues." The blues don't last forever but can cause a rough ten or so days of tears, irritability, anxiety, and fatigue. Then they fade away.

Postpartum depression (PPD) is a different story. One in five mothers experiences mild to serious feelings of depression during pregnancy and in the first year postpartum, and this number is assumed to be low as it often goes unreported. Women are more susceptible to depression during times of transition, especially during their reproductive years. Brain chemistry changes in pregnancy and postpartum are significant, and neurotransmitters, the signals that manage emotion and mental processing, are in states of flux. This means that the mental health changes are physiological, and not due to inadequate or a lack of coping skills.

How do you know if it's a case of the baby blues, or PPD? The first is timing. The baby blues usually stop around two weeks post-birth. PPD can go on for months. Lack of interest in your baby or having difficulty bonding with them, avoiding family and friends, or an inability to take care of yourself or your baby are symptoms to watch for. And if you have suicidal thoughts, cannot stop crying, or consider harming your baby, it's time to get help. Mental health professionals are available in person and via video chat, text, apps, or phone. So are friends and family. Reach out to whomever makes you feel comfortable—but, please, do not ignore these thoughts or resist outside help.

EATING WHILE PARENTING

Gone is the need to avoid deli meat. But now that you're not pregnant, what should you eat? To the surprise of no one, postpartum dietary recommendations are just as varied as those proposed during pregnancy. Warm cooked foods, bone broth, and plenty of protein and iron-rich items that are easy to digest are common to many postpartum nutritional plans. The easiest thing to do: If you developed a sustainable, moderate routine while pregnant, continue to eat the same way. A good framework is eating a mix of lean proteins with whole grains, fresh fruits and vegetables, and dairy, and avoiding processed foods, added sugars, and trans fats.

Immediately after birth is not the time to diet or restrict calories, especially if you are breastfeeding. Breastfeeders have more nutritional and caloric requirements than pregnant women, though similarly, it's a relatively small amount. What you eat goes into breast milk and can shape your child's dietary preferences later. Staying well hydrated is key to helping your body heal and produce breast milk, so drink plenty of water throughout the day, too.

If family and friends offer to pitch in, give them your general dietary guidelines and dishes you like but try not to be too picky. If you're not on the meal train, food delivery services and cooking in large batches ensures you always have things around. Speaking of convenience, healthy snacks are another must in this period, so identify a few items that speak to you and buy them in bulk.

Finally, a note on supplements and vitamins. Many women are prescribed an iron supplement to offset deficiencies caused by bleeding during birth, and postpartum anemia is common. When you attend your postpartum appointment, your ob-gyn or midwife will likely check your levels. If you're taking an iron supplement, know it can cause constipation, and consuming more fiber can help. Eating iron-rich foods is an important way to build back iron stores, but it's not always enough. A multivitamin and mineral complex can be beneficial, and if you are breastfeeding, it's recommended to continue the prenatal vitamins (and yours should contain iron) until you stop.

THE RETURN OF YOUR PERIOD (AND WHAT TO DO ABOUT BIRTH CONTROL)

Sex may be the last thing on your mind right now. But when you do feel ready to give it a try, think about that friend, family member, or celebrity with kids whose birthdays are close together. Like, *really* close, maybe just a single year apart. Though it sounds crazy, you can get pregnant again as soon as ten days after giving birth. Regardless of whether you gave birth via C-section or vaginally, the medical guideline is no sex until six weeks postpartum to allow any tears or scars to heal. When it actually feels right is personal, so be honest with your partner if you're not there yet.

Lactational amenorrhea, or period and ovulation suppression thanks to the high levels of prolactin required for breastfeeding, is why breastfeeding is positioned as birth control. And it's true—if you have not had your period since birth and are exclusively breastfeeding, you probably will not ovulate. But—and it's an important *but*—there are strict rules that you must follow *perfectly* for it to work. Not following them perfectly is how two in one hundred women get pregnant while exclusively breastfeeding in the first six months.

Let's get specific. Exclusive breastfeeding is highly effective birth control only if your baby is receiving no other food, formula, or bottles, and you are nursing at least every four hours during the day and every six hours at night—no pumping. Also important: It only works during the first six months of a baby's life, or until their diet includes real foods. When executed flawlessly, breastfeeding is around 96 percent effective, the same as the pill. When it's not, you'll welcome another baby sooner than you planned. Also important: You can start ovulating before your period returns, so you can't count on that milestone to tell you when to use backup birth control methods.

There are plenty of breastfeeding-approved backup birth control choices. Condoms, diaphragms, and non-hormonal IUDs are all possibilities if you'd rather stay free of extra hormones. The shot, hormonal IUDs, implants, and a pill formulation called the minipill are safe-while-breastfeeding hormone-delivery options. You will not receive formulations that contain estrogen immediately, since it can hurt milk production. Long-acting reversible control options like IUDs can be less painful to insert after birth since your cervix may still be dilated.

When your period comes back is variable and depends on whether you are breastfeeding. Lochia, the postpartum shedding of your baby's well-loved uterine lining, can be confused with the period. It usually lasts around six weeks and lightens over time. But a period can come back as soon as four weeks after birth, or it can take as long as twelve months.

VISITING HOURS

One nice bonus of having a newborn is that everyone comes to you, especially in those early weeks, many times armed with food and presents. Unfortunately, well-meaning, excited friends and family often overstay without considering the stress of hosting while adjusting to life as a new parent. This trend can start in the hospital and go on long after birth.

You and the baby can get partied out quickly, so before you

welcome a parade of people, set expectations. Here are a few things to think about:

- Pediatricians will tell you not to let your guests play hot potato and pass the newborn around, especially if they have germ magnets, a.k.a. toddlers, at home. Be prepared for disappointed faces if you tell someone no.
- If you plan to let someone hold the baby, keep hand sanitizer around or direct your guest to wash their hands before picking them up. Newborn pertussis can be fatal, so make sure anyone holding your newborn received a Tdap vaccine.
- The way your parents or in-laws did things may not be the same way you choose to do things. Seeing them holding or feeding your baby differently can be hard to watch. It's even harder not to correct them. Most of the time, it's better to just let them enjoy their time together, unless they are doing something potentially dangerous (like putting a newborn on their stomach to sleep). If they want to learn or are open to feedback, have at it.
- The opposite can also happen when your guests provide unwelcome commentary about your parenting style. Rather than silently resenting the advice giver, if you are on the receiving end of well-intentioned feedback, smile, say thanks, and let it go.
- Keep visits short. For friends, an ideal visit duration is around thirty minutes. Family and people who are there to lend a hand can stay longer.
- Don't feel like tidying up or hosting? Invite friends for a stroller walk and dose of fresh air.
- If you don't want pictures of your baby (or you) posted on social media, let people know.

The last point isn't just about friends and frenemies seeing your weird postpartum hair (we've all been there, and bad news—it gets worse!). Deciding what and how much to share about your baby online is worth considering sooner rather than later. Posting their birth date, full name, and place of birth can make your baby a future target of identity thieves. Photos can be used by AI to create deepfakes and for other fraudulent purposes too. Then there is the question of consent, which your baby cannot give, and whether your future adult wants photos of them dressed as a cabbage or hatching from an egg discovered by a girlfriend or boss later on.

As a family, we do not post photos of our boys publicly, mostly because we feel their online identity is theirs to own, not ours. Not sharing has its downsides, namely I think they're adorable and they do many outrageous things. We do manage a private shared album to give the grandparents and family their fill.

FEEDING TIME

Newborn nutrition from breast to bottle, and learning to manage that milk production factory

In the early weeks, your baby will eat a lot—between eight and twelve times per day. Why so frequently? Your baby's stomach is really, really tiny at birth. On day one, it can hold a little over one teaspoon of milk and is around the size of a marble. By day three, it's around the size of a Ping-Pong ball. And at one month it is the size of an egg. For comparison, your stomach is around the size of a clenched fist and can expand three to four times its size.

Whether you're breastfeeding or bottle-feeding, meeting your newborn's nutritional needs is a full-time job. Each feeding, which in those first months is every two to three hours, takes twenty to thirty minutes to finish. And the clock on the next feeding doesn't start when your baby has had enough. It starts when the boob or bottle first entered their mouth, meaning at most you'll have around two and a half hours before you do it all again. Beyond managing a hangry baby, if you are breastfeeding, there is a 24/7 milk production facility to manage too.

People have passionate opinions about the right way to feed babies. But rarely does anyone acknowledge the systemic challenges of breastfeeding, or that our world is not designed to support it. One example is the guideline on breastfeeding duration. The official recommenda-tion for new moms who can breastfeed is exclusive breastfeeding for six months and continuing in some form until age two. How work-ing mothers are meant to pull off this feat of time and geographical management is not included in the guideline. Around a quarter of US mothers return to work within two weeks postpartum, so even for those who desperately wish to breastfeed, pumping is the only option. And pumping is not breastfeeding. Breastfeeding is logistically simpler over the long term if you work remotely, have a flexible schedule, or stay home with your baby. But even with freedom, the time and body commitment is a surprise to most first-time moms—even those who love the experience.

If breastfeeding is working well at your house, it's easy to forget that you never know what's going on for other parents. Some deal with a combination of post-birth complications—sleep deprivation, anxiety, or postpartum depression—and need a break from the boob to heal themselves. Breastfeeding at any cost is linked to the onset of postpartum depression and anxiety, which can lead mothers to be less emotionally present—the opposite of breastfeeding's intended effect. There are also issues like tongue-tie, which can impede a baby's abil-ity to latch while also reducing supply. And let's not forget the parents who adopt, have cancer, or use a gestational carrier.

Breastfeeding can be beautiful, but it is not the only way to give your baby a great start in life. Begin your feeding journey with realistic goals, whatever they are, and be flexible as things change. Because, like birth plans, the best-laid breastfeeding ambitions do not always work perfectly. If breastfeeding was smooth with a first child, it may not be the second or third time around, even with the benefit of prior expe-rience. Educate yourself, try what feels right for your family, seek help if you need it, and don't beat yourself up if it isn't working. Whether you choose to exclusively breastfeed, use breast milk in combination with formula, or go with formula only, FED is best.

BREASTFEEDING BREAKDOWN

Breast milk is a fascinating, complex, and highly nutritional substance that we cannot yet replicate exactly in a lab. Breast milk composition adapts as your baby grows and their nutritional requirements change too. Breastfed babies may have a reduced risk of asthma, respiratory infections, SIDS, diabetes, childhood leukemia, eczema, inflammatory bowel disease (IBD), and obesity. Just like what you eat when your baby is in utero, the makeup of breast milk also influences future food preferences and eating behaviors. The skin-to-skin contact supports emotional regulation, giving both of you a hit of oxytocin, too. For moms, breastfeeding decreases the amount of postpartum blood loss and helps the uterus return to its prepregnancy state more quickly. It may also lower the risk of ovarian and breast cancers, high blood pressure, and type 2 diabetes.

However, take note of the word *may* above. Income, education, race, culture, working status, and the presence (or absence) of maternity leave all impact whether a woman breastfeeds and for how long. It is also difficult to control for all confounding factors that impact a child's health and development, and long-term health outcomes for moms. If you can and want to try breastfeeding, you should. But in the spirit of presenting an accurate, holistic view, here is the truth about what you may have heard about breastfeeding for your reading pleasure.

Myth: Breastfeeding comes naturally to everyone

Breastfeeding is a complex dance between a mother and baby that requires patience, persistence, and constant adjustment. C-section moms especially have unique challenges and usually a longer delay until milk comes in. That said, the first days of breastfeeding can be tough even if you had a vaginal birth or your milk is flowing freely, which is why many hospitals employ lactation consultants (LCs).

After you leave the hospital, LCs are available for in-home visits and virtually. If you're using a doula, many can also help with breastfeeding. Here is advice sourced from both groups to get things started:

- Set a timeline goal for how long you'd like to breastfeed, but be flexible if things aren't working.
- Pump from the beginning to stimulate supply (there is nuance here, but it's important for C-section moms).
- Drink water (around sixteen cups (!!!) per day is ideal; keep a water bottle nearby).
- Rest whenever possible.
- Eat a well-rounded diet based on whole foods and follow your body's cues.

Myth: Bigger breasts equal more milk

Good news for all the A and B cups out there: Size has nothing to do with breastfeeding success. The number of ducts inside of a breast is what drives milk production. If you've had a breast surgery, including an augmentation, lift, reduction, or reconstruction, that can influence the nerves and ducts required for milk production. Implants above the muscle, and those that involve the areola and nipple, are especially challenging, as the nerves in the nipple signal your brain to release oxytocin to get milk flowing. How much milk you are able to produce and release depends on how well the nerves and ducts repaired themselves during your recovery.

Myth: Breastfeeding will help you drop all the baby weight

Breastfeeding is touted as a post-birth weight-loss method. And it's true that your caloric burn will be higher if you're breastfeeding. But so will your hunger level. Supply-boosting snacks often close or exceed that deficit, and most women will hold on to the last few pounds of fat (fat helps with milk supply) until the baby is weaned.

But let it be said again: Give yourself some grace and time for your body to recover from the miraculous feat of growing and birthing a human.

Myth: You will make the same amount of milk at every breastfeeding session

Supply must be built from scratch at the beginning of a breastfeeding journey, and it changes based on everything from your baby's demands to your diet and hydration or rest and sleep. Even once your supply is established, you'll need to abide by the same basic rules to keep it. Exclusively breastfed babies are twice as likely as formula-fed babies to be readmitted to the hospital in the first month after birth due to dehydration and jaundice, both of which are signs of underfeeding. The best way to know how much milk you are making is to track soiled diapers (what goes in must go out!). If your baby is overly fussy or seems hungry after every feed, there may be an issue.

Myth: Babies that are breastfed longer have higher IQs

Maybe you heard about a study showing a link between longer breastfeeding duration and higher childhood IQ. What these studies neglect to mention is that maternal IQ is more predictive of a child's IQ than anything else—including race, education, age, economic status, smoking, home environment, birth weight, and birth order—and mothers who breastfeed for longer statistically have higher IQs.

Myth: Breastfeeding gives your baby a supercharged immune system all the way through childhood

Breastfeeding's major health benefits occur in the first few months of life mostly in the form of fewer gastrointestinal issues and rashes. It is not tied to virus-fighting superpowers, does not mean you can skip vaccines, and none of these benefits are proven to extend meaningfully beyond the first six months.

Myth: Breastfeeding happens on the same schedule every day

I can hear the second- and third-time parents chuckling at this one. A strict schedule for a newborn is not a thing. It will take a few weeks for you to find your groove, and between cluster feedings that help stimulate supply and random late-night who-knows-if-it's-day-or-night sessions, it's hard to predict when you'll feed consistently. However, one thing you can do from the beginning is teach a baby what to expect before and after feedings. One example is keeping the environment and skin-to-skin or holds similar. Another way is to follow a consistent routine—wake, change diaper, feed, burp, play, read, nap—each time.

> *Conversations with friends prepared me for the reality that breastfeeding is a full-time job. Stories of mastitis and pumping in closets and leaking breasts and bleeding nipples frankly had me dreading it. On the first point, they were right. I spent a solid eight to ten hours every day in various states of boobs out. But I loved breastfeeding for the months I was able to do it. The time with Mr. Baby was magical. He made adorable happy feeding noises, he snuggled into my chest, and I got high on baby-head smell every session. Pumping, which I had to do to attempt to overcome low supply, was not my favorite. It was messy and inconvenient and made me feel like a cow.*

How breastfeeding works

Newborn feedings are frequent and will be responsive for the first few weeks versus running on a strict timetable. Typically, newborns will need to feed at least every three hours during that time, and yes, you'll have to wake a sleeping baby if yours snoozes through its hunger signals. Feeding cues to follow include rooting (moving their head and mouth around), sucking on fingers, and crying (which is a late sign of hunger).

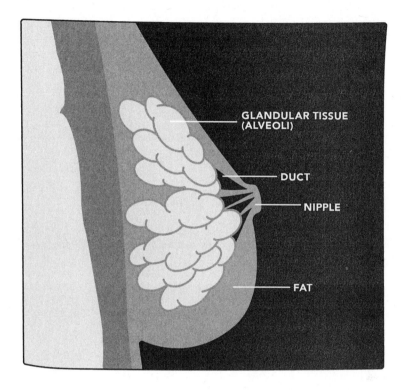

The human breast is made of supporting connective tissue and fat, blood, lymphatic vessels, and nerves, and, relevant to breastfeeding, ducts, mammary tissue, a nipple, and an areola. The rise in estrogen and progesterone levels at the end of the first trimester increases the number of milk ducts in the breasts. The inside of a breast looks like a bunch of grapes, with stem-like ducts, and alveoli, which look like individual grapes. After birth, the ducts transport milk to be released from the nipple.

The two hormones that affect breastfeeding are prolactin and oxytocin. Prolactin is the hormone that signals milk production, and oxytocin, also known as the love hormone, makes the milk flow and fill the ducts. Oxytocin also helps shrink your uterus after birth and is part of the parent/child bonding process.

At the start of each feed, the baby latches to the breast and stretches the nipple while cupping their tongue around the sides beneath the milk ducts. They use suction to press the nipple against their palate, which stimulates the oxytocin reflex and the flow of milk. With a good latch, the baby takes in not just the nipple, but also the areola and surrounding tissue, with a wide-open mouth. The chin should be touching or almost touching the breast, and more of the areola should be visible above the baby's top lip than below the lower lip.

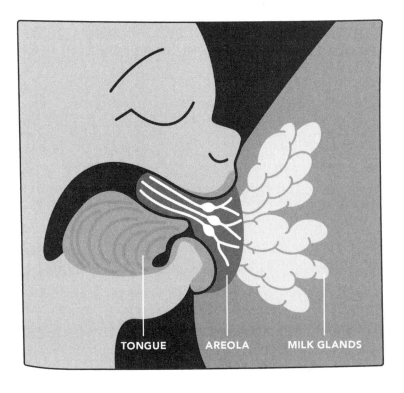

TONGUE   AREOLA   MILK GLANDS

When the latch is right, the suckling can be pleasurable. A bad latch can be painful, and you'll know because it hurts, and your baby will express frustration. If only the nipple is in the baby's mouth, they cannot access the ducts to press and express milk. If you have a bad latch, it's best to try again. Break the latch by gently putting a (clean) pinky into your baby's mouth, hooking it over the top of the nipple, and very gently pulling it away. Then, reposition and try again.

It is hard to see unless you're pumping, but milk doesn't come out of one hole in the nipple, it comes out of several simultaneously. You can see and hear the baby swallow, sometimes pausing to allow the ducts to fill again. Foremilk comes out first and can look thin and watery. The fat-rich hindmilk is released later in a feed as each breast empties. When the baby is satisfied, they will usually pull off on their own. It's important to let them stay on until they let go, as the end of a breastfeeding session is when the hindmilk flows out.

Breastfeeding positions

There are many ways to hold your baby while breastfeeding, so consider these popular options a starting point and experiment. After a vaginal birth, you can take your pick, and it's more a matter of finding what works best for you and your baby. For C-section moms, side-lying and football will help take some pressure off your incision. There are breastfeeding pillows and slings galore if you want to gear up, or you can use a pillow you already own for extra support. The most important positioning criteria are comfort and that your baby can get a good latch, as in those first weeks you'll do this every few hours.

Breastfeeding hunch is real. Even if you reliably switch sides, or swap positions frequently, spending so much time feeding a baby in those first months takes a physical toll on your body. Massage and bodywork is helpful if your partner is willing to step in either to take over baby care so you can get professional help, or to give you frequent shoulder rubs.

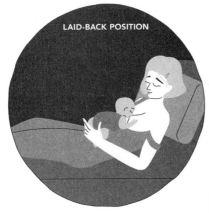

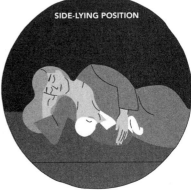

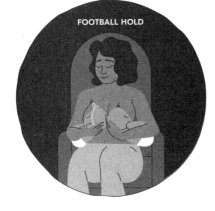

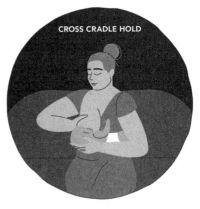

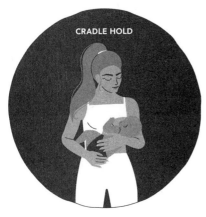

Breastfeeding how-to

You have a few positions to try, so now, here is a quick guide to breast-feeding best practices.

1. **Nose to nipple:** Get your baby in position. Hold their body close and bring their nose level to your nipple while squeezing your breast into a flattened sandwich.
2. **Wide-open mouth:** Tip your baby's head back slightly so their lip brushes your nipple, which should make your baby open wide with their chin touching your breast.
3. **Clear nose; full, round cheeks:** Make sure their nose is not smashed into your breast (read: they can breathe), and that you can see more of your nipple above your baby's top lip than their bottom when they latch. Their cheeks should be round and full as they feed.
4. **Burp and switch sides:** Ten to fifteen minutes into each feed, gently move your baby off the breast, burp them (put your baby on your shoulder and, with a slightly cupped hand, gently pat until you hear a burp), and rotate to the other breast. When your baby finishes, burp them again.

Breast maintenance

Breast maintenance issues and infections can cause speed bumps with feeding, too. Take good care of your breasts with the tips below, and use lanolin or coconut oil to keep your nipples moist and free of cracks.

- **Cleaning:** There is no need to wash your breasts between feedings—letting milk dry on your nipples is fine. When you shower (do it daily), wash your breasts with warm, clear water, and change nursing pads when they become damp or wet.

- **Support:** Wear a bra made of cotton or a breathable blend that is not too tight or too loose. Avoid underwire while you are nursing, and consider buying a few nursing bras in various shades so you never need to take them off. The only exception: There are bras made specifically for pumping that hold the flanges in place so you don't have to. Only caveat is that they don't really work to wear in daily life.

- **Managing pain:** Nipple shields can help during nursing sessions, and there are cushions you can add to pump flanges to make them more comfortable. If you are engorged, gently massage your breast, use warm, moist compresses, or stand in a warm shower. If you experience pain after pumping or nursing, use an ice pack for twenty minutes afterward.

Gauging your milk supply

Breastfeeding is a supply-and-demand operation, so unless you are pumping and giving a bottle, you will not know exactly how many ounces of milk your baby is getting at each feed from each breast. Frustrating, I know.

Tracking diapers is the best overall indicator of how well feeding is going. The first two days, there will be only two to three wet diapers per day and a disturbing-looking meconium poop. But from day four through the first six weeks, you should have at least six wet diapers and two poops (yellow if you're feeding breast milk exclusively; formula turns poop a shade of green—we'll go deep on poop later).

All babies lose weight at birth, but they should be back up to their birth weight within two weeks. More data isn't always better: Unless your baby is premature, your pediatrician asks you to track their weight, or you suspect a problem, weighing a newborn multiple times per day creates more anxiety than it's worth, as their weight fluctuates based on whether they've peed or pooped recently. If you're worried and not already tracking diaper changes, use an app or leave a pad of paper by the changing table for all caregivers to take notes.

On your end, there should not be pain or soreness after the feed. On your baby's, they should feed with a large mouthful of your breast; take long, rhythmic sucks and swallows; and appear content when they pull off the breast at the end of a session. They will let you know if they are still hungry. If they fall asleep on the boob frequently, do a diaper change right before each feed to wake them up, and you can flick or tickle their foot to keep them engaged.

Breastfeeding troubleshooting

Lactation struggles and their remedies are covered in the first known medical encyclopedia, Egypt's Papyrus Ebers, which dates back to 1500 BCE. Wet nurses were frequently utilized in the case of low supply or inability to nurse, up until the 1900s. Creative (sometimes strange) workarounds for breastfeeding challenges included warming the bones of a swordfish in oil and massaging the mother's back with it, and giving her fragrant bread to eat while rubbing her breasts with the poppy plant.

Struggles can be as simple as a bad latch or bad positioning. Insufficient glandular tissue and hypoplasia are known causes of low supply. Hormones and illness can also affect how things go, as can breast surgery. So can not getting enough rest or drinking enough water. There are also medical conditions like mastitis, thrush, and clogged ducts, which are all common but sometimes require medical attention. Mastitis especially can be serious.

Physical issues for your baby can also cause breastfeeding chal-lenges. Tongue-tie—when the tissue anchoring the base of the tongue is too tight—can hurt supply and prevent your baby from getting enough milk at feedings. It affects how the baby moves their tongue, making it difficult for them to latch and stimulate the breast properly to encourage milk production. There is a procedure to fix it called "snipping" (which is exactly what it sounds like), but it is painful and babies can grow out of the issue. Tongue-tie is generally more common in boys than in girls, and sometimes a pediatrician will catch it in the hospital or after you go home, while other times it goes undetected until there is an issue.

Torticollis is another condition that causes a baby's head to rotate or tilt at an awkward angle. We don't really know why it happens, but it's more common in firstborn children and is linked to congenital hip dislocation, perhaps due to the baby's position in the uterus. You'll know if your baby's head tilts to one side constantly. Babies can be born with torticollis or acquire it over time, but either way, early diagnosis followed by physical therapy is the best way to manage it.

There are other feeding challenges that can originate at birth or pop up over time too. These can include difficulty swallowing or rejecting bottles or the breast, or frequently losing liquid from their mouth while drinking. They may wake up one day and decide they hate your breast milk due to something you ate, or no longer like the bottle you've been using. Babies evolve through many phases. Some issues pass or can be treated at home or are solved by swapping dietary choices or equipment, so do not hesitate to reach out to friends or professionals for help if the issues persist or you can't cope.

Mr. Baby had tongue-tie at birth, which meant it could have been challenging for him to latch. Lucky for us, that didn't stop him, perhaps in part because, according to the nurses and LCs, I had "perfect breastfeeding nipples"—the strangest compliment I've ever received.

Breastfeeding tips for C-section moms

There's no way to sugarcoat this: Establishing breastfeeding is usually harder and takes longer after a C-section than a typical vaginal birth. It requires effort, patience, and persistence in those first days. Try skin-to-skin contact as soon as possible after birth, preferably within the first hour when possible (talk to your doctor and put it on your birth preferences). Pump and hand express (have an LC show you how, but yes, it's kind of like milking yourself) and feed on demand (or every two to three hours if your baby is on the sleepy side). Use a breastfeeding pillow and have a nurse or partner hand you the baby and help with positioning. Some hospitals mandate rooming-in, because the more time you spend with your baby, the more likely breastfeeding is to work. However, you just endured major abdominal surgery and need rest. There is no shame in asking someone to take the baby for a walk or to the nursery so you can snatch a few valuable hours of sleep.

Mr. Baby's patience ran out after two days of nothing after birth. I worked with an LC and started a regimen known as the triple feed to stimulate the flow of milk. This involved feeding Mr. Baby, then hand expressing, then pumping, every two to three hours. It was intense. Try as I might, even with a hospital-grade pump, I could coax nothing more than a few tiny beads of colostrum (the nutrient-rich first milk your body makes) out, which I gathered and fed to him with a plastic spoon.

All babies lose weight after birth, but once it exceeded 10 percent, I knew that the hospital would encourage temporary formula supplementation. When the pediatrician told us Mr. Baby's weight was down 12 percent, we agreed to try it. After that first formula feeding with a tiny orange plastic syringe, the screaming stopped, and he finally slept longer than fifteen minutes. I still did all the milk-stimulating things and fed him every drop, but with a little help his weight stabilized, and we got to go home.

On day five postpartum, I woke up after several hours of (finally) unbroken sleep to find myself with comically large, engorged boobs. My milk had arrived. I've always been on the smaller side in that department, so it was a little shocking at first, and then sort of cool.

Dealing with low supply and galactagogues

Today's options to improve breast milk supply go beyond rubbing your body with fish oil or flower petals (but hey, try it if you want!). Since the internet probably knows about your new addition, ads for mysterious supercharged-milk-supply products, or galactagogues, may be rampant in your feeds. Though it sounds more like a way to take your breasts to space, galactagogues are foods, drugs, and herbs that are supposed to increase breast milk production. And over half of mothers report using them.

There is no clinical evidence that, beyond a placebo effect, galactagogues make a real difference. Trials to date have not been well controlled or have small sample sizes. LCs recommend trying repositioning, more frequent pumping, breast compression, and skin-to-skin first. In more extreme cases, there are also prescription medications that can boost milk supply.

Anecdotally, people swear by these mega-milk-producing substances. If you want to give them a shot, fenugreek, alfalfa, blessed thistle, goat's rue, and moringa are the top herbal supplement picks and primary ingredients in mother's-milk tea, tinctures, and bars. Chat with your doctor to ensure they don't cause side effects or interactions with other medications you're taking. Those that are not foods are classified as supplements, which are largely unregulated and will not have much, if any, safety information.

Eating specific foods is another route to increased supply. The most commonly cited milk boosters are almonds, anise, barley, brewer's yeast, chickpeas, coconut, dill, millet, oats, and rice. All of these are nutritious and fine to mix into your daily routine.

Another less nutritious but popular solution for low production is beer. One of the polysaccharides in the barley used to make beer seems to stimulate prolactin. Drinking a single beer right after a feeding or pumping session is best, as it takes around two hours to clear out of your bloodstream and breast milk. But don't overdo it—alcohol reduces production, so one is enough.

We still don't know how many women have low supply and why. If you've tried everything, are pumping and hand expressing around the clock, have worked with an LC (or two), are eating your weight in brewer's yeast and oatmeal bars, and nothing is happening, you may want to consider plan B.

Yes, my milk did eventually come in. But even with constant pumping, feeding on demand, hydrating, and trying every imaginable milk-boosting brew, my supply never kept up with Mr. Baby's hunger level. He left every session frustrated, especially on my lazy left boob, which he despised. When I spoke to my panel of experts, they suggested that it could be due to the extra medications and higher than normal blood loss I experienced during birth and resulting anemia.

After twelve weeks of combo feeding, Mr. Baby started screaming every time I put him up to a boob. I transitioned to exclusively pumping, but he also refused to drink that milk, even mixed with formula. The only real theory anyone had was that my breast milk was high in lipase (an enzyme that helps babies digest the natural fats in breast milk), which made it taste and smell metallic or soapy. He refused it even when we mixed it with solids later.

When my second son was born, I followed the same stimulate-supply routine. But despite Herculean effort and frantic sessions with LCs, those engorged boobs never popped. Theories include missing labor hormones, since this time it was straight to a C-section, or that we were separated due to complications on both sides right after birth. But really, I'll never know for sure. At first, I was devastated that my breastfeeding ambitions were dashed again. But I made my peace when I watched him grow from a tiny five-pound peanut to major chunker in a few months on a great formula.

Both of my kids are healthy, have strong immune systems, and devour just about everything I put in front of them—and some things I don't. Toddlers eat food off the floor in public places and lick playground equipment, so at some point as a parent, you realize there's only so much you can do. I'm glad I did all I could with breastfeeding, and also that I listened to the many professionals who kindly told me it was time to stop. As one pediatrician said, there are many ways to show up as a parent, and if anxiety related to breastfeeding was preventing me from showing up as my best self, that mattered, too.

GET PUMPED UP

If you can't be with your baby 24/7, or if breastfeeding isn't working, you may decide to pump your breast milk. It can also be a useful tool in establishing and boosting milk supply. We already covered how to select a breast pump model, but here's a refresher. Insurers are required to provide one gratis, so contact them to explore your options and order. There are new hands-free models that make the job easier, but insurance doesn't pay for them, and they are generally less powerful. Most pumps require holding the flanges in place or use of a pumping bra, as the seal is not strong enough to avoid leakage on its own. On that note, pumping requires accessories, and the internet is there for it. Many of them, from bags to coolers to cover-ups, are stylish and discreet.

The process of pumping is, well, strange. You'll finally understand what it feels like to be a dairy cow and will get used to the gentle rhythmic *whoosh whoosh whoosh* and the hypnotic look of your nipples expanding and squirting streams of milk from tiny holes you didn't know existed. You'll pump the most milk in the morning, when your breasts are fullest, especially once your baby sleeps more than a few hours at a time. You can also pump the other breast during a feed to help your milk flow more easily or use a manual pump to catch that extra milk.

Whether you're out and about, at work, or just at home, here are the top mom-approved pumping tips and tricks:

- Keep an extra set of flanges and pump parts at work and store them in a plastic bag in the refrigerator or cooler. This way, you only clean up once per day and the drips are contained.
- Button-down shirts make pumping and breastfeeding speedier. Your breastfeeding cover-up works to keep things undercover, too.
- Carry an extra shirt or paper towels to help with unexpected leakage and drips.
- Having trouble with letdown? Look at photos or a video of your baby or carry a onesie that smells like them.
- Slather on the nipple cream to keep things moist before and after pumping. Many are baby-friendly, so you won't have to wash it off if you're still nursing.
- Consider keeping a manual hand pump around. They're cheap and easy to use on the go.
- Buy back-up parts for your pump, and keep them clean, especially the tiny plastic membranes, which can easily go down the drain while washing.
- If you don't have access to a refrigerator to store milk or room to store a mini model at your desk, tote a cooler with ice packs from home.
- Though you'll have to pay for it, consider buying a second pump that just lives at work, especially if you take public transportation.

What do you do with all this extra milk? Freeze it, baby. Getting a stash going is great before you go back to work, for the times you won't be with your baby, and in case your supply drops. When you bag it up, label it with the date pumped, and store in varying amounts so nothing goes to waste—for example, one-ounce and two-ounce bags are useful if your production unexpectedly drops and you need a top-off, whereas a four-ounce bag can get you through a whole feeding. Mind the bag's fill lines, since milk expands while freezing.

Pumped milk stays good at room temperature for four hours, in a refrigerator for up to three days, in your normal freezer for six months, and in a deep freezer for up to twelve months. When you are ready to thaw, breast milk can be stored in the refrigerator for up to twelve hours, or you can hold it under warm running water to use more quickly. Never use the microwave or boiling water, as they can damage breast milk's nutritional properties. And when that liquid gold finally goes into the bottle, think swirled, not shaken, if the fat has separated.

WEANING

You may not be there right now, but at some point, your breastfeeding journey with this baby will come to an end. Regardless of why you are stopping or when, weaning gradually is the way to avoid engorgement, discomfort, and mastitis. This means targeting dropping one feeding every three to seven days, depending on how things go to allow your supply to drop slowly. Weaning at day and at night also require different strategies. However, when you decide it's time, consider booking a session with an LC (virtually is fine) to devise a plan as the process and how it plays out is nuanced.

If you're reading and dreaming of a full night's sleep, night weaning requires a slightly different approach and should not be done while you try to wean during the day. There is no right time to stop breastfeeding at night, as every baby is different. But a few key tactics: Maximize feeds during the day and keep distractions to a minimum; consider dream feeding (nursing two or three hours after they go down for bed with minimal stimulation) to stretch their fullness; and try nursing from only one breast at bedtime, then the other breast during a dream feed or when the baby wakes so they access the high-fat hindmilk. If things aren't going well, your baby may not be ready to wean, or they could be teething or going through another developmental milestone that interferes with their sleep.

For daytime weaning, begin by slowly shortening the feed that is least critical for your baby, or, if they're older than six months, try dropping it entirely. Last to go will be sessions before naps, bedtime, and first thing in the morning. Extra cuddle sessions and snuggles can help with the loss of physical contact during breastfeeding, and if there is a new fear of separation or other signs of distress, consider slowing things down. With older babies and toddlers, LCs suggest the "don't offer, don't refuse" approach. Distraction is your friend. Plan your day so you're out doing something that they enjoy during that feed, like a trip to the playground, and provide a different snack. You can also use it as a first lesson in patience and tell them "not now."

BOTTLE-FEEDING BASICS

Whether it's pumped milk so your partner can pitch in with feedings, or if you're combo feeding and supplementing with formula or exclusively formula feeding, you'll spend a lot of time thinking about—and washing—bottles. If you are transitioning from breast to bottle, it can happen right after birth, or months into your feeding journey when it's time to go back to work.

Introducing a bottle to a breastfed baby can take a few attempts, but there are a few ways to optimize the likelihood of success. The first time you offer a bottle, have someone else (not the breastfeeding mother) give it to them, at a time your baby is relaxed and not too hungry. Doing skin-to-skin to simulate the closeness of breastfeeding can help, as can trying positions that you don't usually use during breastfeeding sessions. Keeping the number of people who feed your baby small at first can also help bottle feeding stick.

All babies, even those who stubbornly reject bottles at first, will eventually take one with enough persistence. If you're going back to work, start the bottle transition process a few weeks before you're due back, as it can take time. Sometimes physical therapy is needed if there is an issue that requires treatment. If you're having trouble, speak to your pediatrician or to an LC.

Choosing bottles and navigating nipples

A key difference between breastfeeding and bottle feeding is how quickly and consistently milk flows. It's hard work to pull milk out of a breast; bottles are easy in comparison, which means you must choose the right flow rate on the nipple.

There are many, many bottle options: low-flow, fast-flow, vented, glass, plastic, silicone, flat or natural nipples—the list goes on. Human breasts expel milk from several holes, and some brands follow a similar design to mimic this process, starting with tiny holes and expanding their size as your baby grows. Others, known as variable-rate nipples, respond to the pressure your baby applies, allowing them to control how much milk flows. And still others increase the number of holes with age to allow more milk to pass. As with every other accessory, it comes down to your baby's preferences, so have a few options on hand. To get you started, for a gassy or colicky baby, a low-flow or vented bottle is a good choice. For a baby who loves the boob, try a breast-like nipple. Pumping frequently? Find a container that doubles as a bottle so you can pump, screw on the nipple, and feed.

Every time you try a new bottle, you'll need to sterilize it and all the nipples, caps, and rings by boiling them in hot water for at least ten minutes, or by using a sterilizing solution or steam unit. The first three months are when your baby's immune system is the weakest, so keeping bottles clean and sterile is most important during that phase. Unless your baby was premature or has a weakened immune system, washing them well with hot water and soap is fine after that time. Let them dry completely before using.

Bottle-feeding quick-start guide

If you're using formula, follow the directions on the package to prepare your bottle. For powders, mix with boiling water and allow it to cool. Test the temperature by squirting a few drops on your wrist before offering. If it is too hot, run the bottle under cold water to cool it down. Never add sugar or cereal or extra formula to a bottle to attempt to fill your baby up—it's not a thing. If you're reheating breast milk, put the bottle into a container of hot water or run it under hot water—do not use the microwave. Fresh-expressed milk can be served cold, and frozen breast milk can be thawed in advance in the refrigerator before using, then prepared using the method above. Some babies are fine with their bottles on the cool side, while others prefer it warm. Once you find their preference, consistency from feeding to feeding is helpful.

Paced feeding is an ideal way to start offering a bottle, as it puts your baby in charge of how much milk they need and allows for breaks, reducing the likelihood of overfeeding, gas, and spit-up. It requires a slow-flow nipple and a small bottle that holds between four and five ounces. You'll start by positioning your baby semi-upright (versus a reclined or cradle hold) with the bottle held parallel to the ground so that milk flows slowly.

1. Tickle their lips with the nipple and allow them to latch on deeply, keeping the bottle horizontal.
2. Once they establish a strong latch, tilt the bottle up slightly so milk begins to flow. Let them get between three and five swallows (this should take around thirty seconds), then tilt the bottle back down to the horizontal position.
3. Repeat this process for ten to fifteen minutes, burp, and then switch sides (same as you would do during

breastfeeding so they build neck strength on both sides).

4. If they are pushing the bottle out of their mouth or no longer sucking, milk is leaking out of their mouths, or they splay fingers and toes, those are signs they are full.

5. When finished feeding, burp your baby a final time.

At first, paced feeding may take longer than a typical breastfeeding session, but over time bottle feedings will get faster. Ensure you communicate this process to anyone feeding your baby, whether it's a partner, childcare professional, or family so they follow it, too.

FORMULA

Formulas have come a long way. The first commercial version—a mix of wheat flour, malt flour, cow's milk, and bicarbonate of potash (a salt that contains potassium)—concocted by German chemist Justus von Liebig hit the market in 1869. Experiments followed, and it wasn't until modern formula launched to much fanfare in the 1950s that it was safe, filling, and nutritionally complete enough to truly work for infants. The result: Formula was all the rage, and by 1972, only 22 percent of babies were breastfed.

Then, in 1974, the infamous Baby Killer report was published. It detailed the shady promotion and sales of formula in developing countries and triggered a mass boycott. A few years later, in 1981, there were more than sixty-six thousand infant formula–related deaths in low- and middle-income countries, caused by mixing powdered formula with contaminated water. Even though the problem wasn't the formula powder, it reinvigorated women's interest in breastfeeding, and formula is still sometimes met with suspicion.

We're far beyond potash these days, and companies are working on versions that very closely simulate breast milk. Ingredient-wise, formula contains the same basic vitamins and nutrients as breast milk but lacks the latter's rich antibodies. Most formulas are based on cow's milk or soy milk, which require processing to meet the needs of human infants and are iron-fortified—an ingredient not found in breast milk.

Choosing a good formula isn't straightforward, as much of what makes a formula good for your baby is what works for their specific digestive system. Their preferences and needs can change over time, and you may use more than one.

There is a perception that, like croissants and wine, European formula is better because there is more stringent regulation, and the ingredients are cleaner. That idea is not entirely without merit as: (1) all formulations are organic, since the EU dictates that there are no detectable levels of pesticide residue in formula; (2) the cows are all grass-fed and live on biodynamic farms; and (3) corn syrup is not an ingredient. If you do choose a European formula, pay attention to the stage it's meant for, as the nutrition is tailored to specific age ranges, and ensure you have a good label translation (unless your German is better than mine) so you know what you're getting. Because they aren't FDA-approved and there is counterfeiting (only purchase from trusted sources), your pediatrician may not be amped about a European formula, so be prepared to make your case if it comes up. There are great brands that are made in the US that have most of the same features as European brands, and you'll know exactly where they came from.

Formula comes in three types: powder, concentrated liquid, and ready-to-use. Powder is the easiest for travel, and the cheapest, but can cause constipation and is harder for newborns to digest. You'll need to mix it with water before feeding your baby. Concentrated is more expensive than powder, and still requires added water. Ready-to-use is the priciest but is best for infants with picky digestive systems. Instead of buying huge containers, ask your pediatrician for recommendations. Try each type for at least three days before rejecting it as an option, as it takes time for your baby's digestive system to adjust.

Donor milk

"Liquid gold," they call it. And at $3 to $5 per ounce, the name is fitting. There is a whole regulated industry around donor breast milk for people who need a bridge to breastfeeding or just do not want to use formula. It relies on mothers who have extra production and a milk bank to receive, process, and redistribute the milk. Here's how it works.

To donate at a licensed bank, mothers are given a health screening, including a blood test to ensure they don't have any diseases like HIV or hepatitis that can be transferred to the baby. If approved, the donor pumps and freezes the extra supply (most banks will take deep-frozen milk up to six months after it's pumped) and ships it to the bank in a cooler. The bank then puts the donor milk through a process called Holder pasteurization (HoP). During HoP, the breast milk is slowly unfrozen and heated to 62.5 degrees Celsius for half an hour. The milk is then tested for any pathogens, bacteria, or viruses before it is refrozen and distributed to families in need.

HoP is used around the world to make human milk safe for infants, but there is a downside, namely that the process lowers the concentration of many vitamins (vitamin C is eliminated entirely), as well as fat. It also reduces lactoferrin, a protein that binds iron, which can fight germs and is thought to stimulate intestinal development. Some studies show that HoP has such an impact that families might be better off just using a high-quality formula.

Insurers will cover the cost of donor milk for preemies, especially if they are high-risk or have a very low birth weight, but otherwise, most parents pay out-of-pocket. A one-month-old baby can drink thirty ounces of breast milk per day, and at today's prices, exclusively using donor milk means your tab will be thousands of dollars per month.

Inevitably, the high cost of licensed-donor milk means there is a gray market and a cottage industry of mothers who sell or donate directly. Though it's not technically illegal, if you are considering this even with close friends or family, you should know the risks. There is no guarantee that what you'll receive ordering online is human milk. You won't know with certainty the donor's health history or lifestyle, if she's been exposed to any harmful bacteria or other substances, or what, if any, medications will be passed to your baby. Even with the most well-intentioned donors, this contamination can happen accidentally from poor storage or sterilization methods.

YOUR NEW ROOMMATE

A basic introduction to that brand-new tiny human

We'll get back to you shortly. But since it's a major part of your new existence as a parent, you probably have questions about that adorable baby. Speaking of adorable, ever wonder why babies are so cute? Answer: Cuteness is critical to their survival.

Human babies are completely helpless at birth. And just like we don't know what triggers labor, we don't really understand why they are born at such a deficit. To give a sense of how underdeveloped a newborn human's brain is compared to other primates, to match the cognitive development of a newborn chimpanzee, human gestation would need to be between eighteen and twenty-one months. Functioning as a human is a learned skill, and newborns are unable to communicate their needs in a language more nuanced than whining, cooing, and howling. To decipher these cries for help, it's useful to understand what their post-uterus world is like.

For a while, a newborn is nostalgic for their cozy home in your belly and needs help feeling secure and protected. After nine months of going everywhere with you, motion makes them feel soothed, which means a lot of rocking, walking, swinging, and jiggling. Their behavior beyond crying and sleeping includes burps, hiccups, curling into the fetal position, snuffles, and pauses between breaths for uncomfortable periods of time.

Preference for a tight, womb-like environment aside, what about a baby's senses—hearing, seeing, and tasting?

Newborns know their mother's voice straightaway, as they've heard it over and over during pregnancy. They emerge with decent auditory skills, though the fluid in their middle ear makes them most responsive to high-pitched voices—hence their love of baby talk. Other favorite newborn sounds mimic the *shhhhh*s and gurgles of the womb, which is why white noise and shushing are such popular ways to put babies at ease (or to sleep!).

Their visual abilities are not great for a few months. Newborns can see only up to two feet for the first weeks, and everything looks like a black-and-white movie. Bright lights can cause screaming, so it's wise to keep them out of direct sun. The occasionally cross-eyed gazes deep into your eyes happen because babies LOVE faces. Their second-favorite visuals are high-contrast black-and-white patterns and pictures, as they can't detect color until around four months.

There's nothing on the menu but breast milk or formula for a while, but babies still come loaded with taste preferences. Sweet trumps bitter, and newborns turn away from smells and tastes they don't like. What you ate while pregnant and eat now if you're breastfeeding can influence their eventual flavor and food preferences later. So if you want to optimize the odds that your kid has an adventurous palate, start now by embracing a diverse (but not gas-causing) diet.

Newborns have a hard time regulating body temperature, so dress them in one more layer than you would wear so they are cozy and warm. Initially, most babies HATE being naked, and will scream when undressed or bathed and during diaper changes. While it's natural to try hacks like wipe warmers to get through this loud and painful period, long-term it's easier to power through until they learn to adjust.

The weird umbilical cord stump will dry up and eventually fall off up to a month after birth. In the meantime, keep the area clean and fold your baby's diaper down so it stays dry and heals. Tummy time should wait until after the cord drops off.

Now that we know how they see the world, let's learn more about their primary activities. No matter how unique your baby grows to become, infants are limited to sleeping, crying, eating, and soiling diapers for those first months.

SLEEPING

Newborns spend eight to ten hours during the day sleeping, and six to eight hours at night (though not consecutively for a while), waking mostly to be fed, burped, and put back down for a nap. They do not emerge from the womb understanding the difference between day and night. In fact, most newborns get the two confused at first, which you may have noted at 3:00 a.m. if yours is ready to party. One sleeping pro tip is to make the room where they are napping dark even during the day so they associate dark with sleep. If it's time to play, make sure it's in a light place. And though it's tempting to talk to them at all times, if a nap or bedtime is happening soon, better to stay quiet and let them relax.

Babies who are ready for sleep may tip you off with a yawn, or by rubbing their eyes, looking away from you, or fussing. It can be irresistible to breastfeed or rock a baby all the way to sleep. However, babies who rely exclusively on a parent or boob to go down may have a hard time going back to sleep if they wake up. It's why pediatricians recommend letting a baby get sleepy and calm in your arms but putting them into their crib still awake. A bedtime routine can also be beneficial, as it teaches your baby what to expect. At first it probably won't be much—changing a diaper, feeding, and putting them down to sleep. Eventually it can grow to include reading a book or playing soft, calm music as they settle down at night. A white-noise machine can be helpful early on, especially if it has the librarian setting ("shhh shhh shhh").

There are a lot of rules when it comes to where and how newborns sleep, and many practices are still debated. In 1992, the American

Academy of Pediatrics (AAP) made the "back-to-sleep" recommendation, which advocates that babies sleep on their backs exclusively. It advises against soft surfaces, loose bedding, stuffed toys, blankets, and crib bumpers. Since its publication, the rate of SIDS has dropped more than 50 percent.

While newborn co-sleeping is convenient, and many parents do it, the AAP advises against it for many of the same reasons relating to SIDS. The crib or bassinet should be in the same room, preferably near your bed, for the first six months. But as nice as baby snuggles can be, all sleep is advised to happen separately. This also means that if you have multiples, each baby gets their own sleeping quarters.

How long it takes for a baby to sleep through the night varies based on the baby, but by four months, they can learn how to self-soothe and fall back to sleep on their own. Four months is also the earliest it's recommended to sleep train if you choose to. Ironically, cutting nap time during the day does not help sleep duration at night. Babies who do not get enough rest during the day become overtired and have a harder time staying asleep later.

Swaddling

The involuntary, spastic shooting out of arms and legs has a name: the Moro, or startle, reflex. It is believed to be a primitive survival instinct that alerts the newborn to a loss of balance, which keeps them from losing grip on their mother. It happens randomly and is triggered by a change from one surface to another, unexpected loud noises and changes in light, and anything else that shifts the amount of support they feel. The Moro reflex persists until babies are three to four months and causes fits of crying and can get in the way of sleep. Swaddling is one of the most effective ways to counteract it, as it provides consistent physical support.

Unless you're really good at origami, swaddling perplexes most first-time parents, especially when learning on a squirmy newborn. It may take several tries to find a technique and swaddle that works, depending on how much your baby enjoys jailbreaking. There are different folding methods of varying complexity, and many, many models and materials on the market, including sleep sack swaddles that require little more than putting it on your baby like pj's and securing the Velcro straps. If you do want to try the traditional muslin or cotton blanket folding method, here is the classic diamond swaddle how-to.

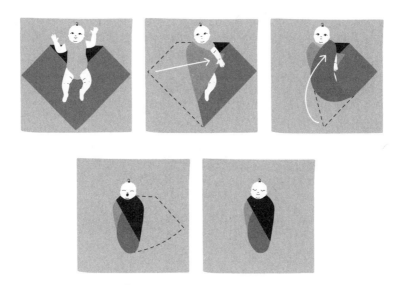

If your baby resists, swaddling may not be for them, as it's meant to provide comfort, not be a punishment. Swaddles should not be used in overly hot climates, or on babies who co-sleep, have a higher risk of SIDS, or have hip issues. As soon as your baby starts rolling over, it's time to take them out of the swaddle. At that point, there may be a sleep regression due to the wildly flapping arms, so consider transitioning slowly, by reducing usage and leaving one arm out during the daytime so they can get used to it before you take it away at night.

A few of Mr. Baby's many nicknames were "little wizard" and "little mage," as his arm flapping made it look like he was casting spells on all who passed. Swaddling worked well for him, though it took five different versions to find one that he couldn't break out of. When he hit eight weeks, he started rolling, so swaddling had to go. And with it went his long-ish spans of sleep at night, as his flailing limbs woke him up.

CRYING

Babies cry for a few reasons: They're hungry, there is a poopy diaper, they are overstimulated, or they hate you. Just kidding! Even if they scream in your face constantly, your baby does not hate you. Crying is their only real way of communicating. Given a little time, you'll understand the difference between whines and *I'm mad* and *Something is seriously wrong.* Promise.

Let's pause for a moment on overstimulation, since it can be tricky to identify. Overstimulation, or letting your baby go into sensory overload from bright light, too much handling, or staring at something for too long, can stand in the way of developing good sleep habits, and lead to loud, tearful screams. When babies wake up from a sleep cycle, they enter into what is known as a quiet alert phase and can stare at objects and take in what's happening around them. Next is active alert, when they are moving and responding to sounds and visuals. Then, the worst phase—when they cry.

Some babies also have what's called a "witching hour," or a specific time of day when they seem to cry for no reason. It's most common toward the end of the day, when body temperature is at its peak and your baby is tired, making it tough to relax. Babies make very little melatonin in the first three months of life when this inexplicable crying peaks; this also contributes, since melatonin is responsible for regulating our sleep/wake cycles.

How do you stop a baby from crying? First, identify the problem. If a baby is hungry, crying is actually a late sign, and they might refuse the boob or bottle. Crying during a feeding? Try burping. Pumping legs accompanied by screaming usually means gas, which can be relieved by bicycling their legs. A reliable way to calm a baby down is to go for a walk, as the fresh air can help them relax. Appealing to their love of sucking is another, hence the popularity of pacifiers.

And then there's colic. It's a condition with no known cause (or at least not one that adults understand) that causes crying for hours and hours at a time. You can identify colic using the rule of three: more than three hours of crying per day for more than three days per week for at least three weeks. It usually peaks around six to eight weeks and improves as babies hit three or four months.

If you reach a breaking point during a never-ending spell of crying, take a breather. Ask your partner to take over, or just put the baby down in a safe place like a crib until you can get it together. It's normal to have these moments; just remember, it won't last forever.

Yes, I googled "Does my baby hate me?" after one particularly epic crying jag. Turned out Mr. Baby did not hate me, he just had really bad gas.

SANITATION DUTY

Newborns can create up to ten dirty diapers per day. The majority are just wet, but one will likely be poopy. Don't be surprised when you crack open a diaper right after birth and find a disturbing greenish-black, sticky, tar-like substance. It's called meconium, and within a few days, it will transition to a more normal-looking color. Breastfed-baby poop has a mustardy texture and can range in hue from classic yellow to seeded Dijon. It smells sweet and can be loose and watery. Formula-fed-baby poop has a peanut-buttery, solid consistency with a more offensive bouquet and ranges from pale yellow to green or light brown. Enjoy the lack of foul odor while you can—once they start eating solid foods, it's all downhill in the smell department.

Colors that deviate from this palette may indicate something is wrong. If the poop is green and watery or slimy, it may be a sign of dehydration or a virus. Dry or hard pellets can indicate constipation. And it's time to call the doctor if there is any pink or red. Though it could be blood the infant swallowed from cracked nipples, it can also mean a milk allergy, an infection, or a rectal tear. Same for thick and black after the first few days of meconium, unless you are using iron-fortified formula.

When you're putting on a diaper, be sure it is well sealed, put on straight, and higher in the back than the front to avoid blowouts. Worried about diaper rash? Make sure your baby's butt is dry and clean after every change. Oh, one more unavoidable thing. If you have a boy, more than once, a tiny stream of urine will hit you in the face or soak your clothes. To limit the number of golden showers, use the soiled diaper as a shield between you and his penis while you lift his butt up and slide the new one on.

Every parent has a poop story—here's ours. The morning after we were discharged from the hospital, I blearily handed Mr. Baby to Nick to change before our first pediatrician visit so I could shower. Limping the four blocks to our appointment took longer than expected, so we were late. This did not surprise the pediatrician, who asked us cheerily to undress Mr. Baby and lay him on the table for an exam. Nick carefully lifted him out of the car seat and blanched. The pediatrician peered over and choked back a laugh. Mr. Baby had used our slow stroll to have a nice, relaxing, shockingly voluminous poop. Unfortunately for him, when sleep-deprived Nick swapped his clothes, he forgot to put on a diaper. Mr. Baby, his onesie, the car seat, and the swaddle were coated in disgusting yellow blowout.

PERCENTILES AND MILESTONES

Figuring out sleeping, eating, crying, and bowel movements will keep you plenty busy in the first months. But another thing that may occupy your mind, especially in those pediatrician appointments, is how your baby is growing and developing.

Ultrasounds during pregnancy were the first time you encountered percentiles for height, weight, and head circumference. And now that your baby is out of the womb, you'll encounter them again at well-baby appointments. The pediatrician will take these measurements and plot them on a chart. Where they fall on that chart compared to other babies of the same age dictates the percentile. If your baby's weight falls in the sixtieth percentile, it means 40 percent of babies at that age weigh more and 60 percent weigh less. What matters more than being too far toward either end of the spectrum is that your baby's growth follows a curve and continues at a steady, predictable rate over time.

Developmental milestones are another way of evaluating how your baby is progressing. Less than half of pediatricians use them in appointments, as they are not a foolproof way of identifying issues. In fact, the four most used developmental checklists are pretty inconsistent. While each list features at least 170 milestones, only forty are common to all four lists, and barely half of those have the same target age for each milestone. For example, one list expects a child's ability to dress and undress to happen at thirty-six months. On another, it's not until month sixty.

Not mapping precisely to these milestones causes a lot of anxiety for parents. And it shouldn't. They are meant to be long-term goals and averages, so try to focus on the big picture.

FINDING YOUR PARENTING STYLE

Cages suspended from the sides of buildings were believed to be an acceptable way to ensure 1930s babies got enough fresh air. And there is almost certainly something your parents or grandparents did that you would not dream of doing with your child (like putting babies to sleep on their stomachs). So it's safe to say that parenting trends come and go. How you choose to raise your baby is a decision only you and your partner can make. But since it's no doubt on your mind, here is a quick overview of common parenting frameworks.

Diana Baumrind, a developmental psychologist, in the 1960s, or-ganized parenting styles based on variances in communication, nur-turance, expectations, and discipline styles. Authoritarians are high on expectations and low on flexibility and use punishment to enforce desired behavior. Permissive parents let their kids do what they want, are warm and nurturing, and often act more like friends than like parents. Uninvolved parents are just that—they give a lot of latitude to their kids and stay out of the way, sometimes due to lack of interest, or because they are just unsure of what to do. Authoritative parents are direct about expectations, clear communicators, nurturing, and include their children in goal- and decision-making. Most research shows that authoritative parenting is the most beneficial style of these options.

So-called gentle parenting also goes by "respectful," "mindful," or "intentional" parenting and is all about fostering the qualities you'd like in your child through compassion and consistency. Its four pillars are empathy, understanding, boundaries, and respect. While it isn't quite as well-honed as Baumrind's archetypes, it rests on the notion that understanding why a child is acting a particular way or even nar-rating their behavior is more effective than a raised voice. Giving a time-out or grounding a child is strictly verboten with this method, as the goal is to teach emotional regulation instead of punishing kids when they get out of control, though there are many derivatives.

The siren song of European child-rearing methods promising perfectly behaved kids in restaurants also may have piqued your in-terest, so let's take a peek at the stereotypical guidelines of French parenting:

- **No means no.** Be consistent in your discipline and let your child know who is in charge.
- **Self-play and independence.** Your child should be able to entertain him- or herself at times, and not lose it every time your attention is elsewhere.
- **Make time for adults.** Spending time with others who are not your child means a more balanced family where your child doesn't think they are the center of the universe.
- **Teach patience and keep a schedule.** No interruptions, stay on a consistent eating schedule, and wait your turn.
- **Eat what the family eats.** No special kid's meals.
- **No baby talk.** Talk to your kids with the same tone of voice you would your partner, and in the same language.

Whether you disagree with the French, or don't identify exactly with any of this, as with pregnancy, and birth, what's most important is finding a parenting style that feels right for your family. If you do it all again, you'll find that what works for a first child often doesn't for the second. The babies will be different humans, and you will come to the experience as a more seasoned parent. You also don't have to adhere to one parenting style—most people end up utilizing a combination of methods and adjusting on the fly.

Here is my n=1 experience as a mom of two very different boys. Mr. Baby has big feelings, and my second could not be more easygoing. They came out of the womb that way, and parenting requires individual approaches and constant adjustment. While I try to always respond with calm, let's be real—we all have hard days, and sometimes it's hard to endure tantrums with perfect cool. Parenting is humbling. My focus is creating safe boundaries, connection, consistency, and repair when needed. You may be a few years off from dealing with toddlers, but it's never too early to take a deep breath and give yourself a break. The newborn months are disorienting and can shake your confidence as a person and a parent—we've all been there.

I am a (very) data-driven person, but I try not to let childhood development studies drive every single parenting decision. If you think pregnancy research is bad, this area is far worse, as findings are frequently dominated by confounding factors or later disproven. Obsessing over every minuscule decision, especially as a first-time parent, usually ends in anxiety or analysis paralysis. Worse, it leads us to ignore our intuition, which lets us simply listen and connect and be present with our kids. At some point, you have to put the books and parenting experts and influencers aside and parent from your gut and heart.

TRANSITIONS

Becoming a parent, mom guilt, returning to work,
and what to think about when you're
ready to do it all again

Becoming a parent is, for most people (especially those who begin the process in their mid-to-late thirties), the biggest personal transformation of our lives. And it doesn't always line up with the image we have in our heads. Maybe you secretly wanted a girl but got a boy. Perhaps you fantasized about bonding during breastfeeding, but that same son won't latch and you have to pump and bottle-feed. Your dreams of being surrounded by friendly moms may be dashed by someone's judgment about your need to bottle-feed. And when you share with your partner, perhaps they don't say the right thing to make you feel better.

Once you get the all-clear from your doctor to resume physical activity, your wavering confidence might get in the way of enjoying the things you used to do. Whether that's yoga or having sex, your relationship with your body is different. Balancing your baby, your partner, work, and yourself (never mind a social life) now happens in the tiny windows between feedings and naps. And it can be hard to express any ambivalence you may be feeling about your new role as a parent to friends and colleagues—it's *supposed* to be a happy time, right? After all, you have a new baby! You're a MOM. Isn't it all delightful and great?

337

Yes. And no.

The transition to motherhood involves obvious physical and lifestyle changes, but there is a lot going on in that mind of yours, too. We know that it takes around two years after birth for your brain to go back to its prepregnancy size. But that's not where the gray-matter changes end. The stereotypical mothering behaviors like fierce protectiveness, worry, and love for your baby have neurological roots. And that hamster wheel in your head telling you over and over to make sure the baby is breathing while they sleep or that worries about leaving them at home with someone who isn't you can be hard to stop. Infertility patients often put tremendous pressure on themselves as new parents since it took so much work, time, and money to make that baby happen; as a result, they experience higher-than-average rates of anxiety.

This identity shift to mother is known as *matrescence*, and it involves physical changes to your brain. The amygdala is an almond-shaped set of neurons deep in the brain's medial temporal lobe that drives emotional reactions and processes memory. Amygdala activity is higher in the months after childbirth and drives mothering behaviors by making you more sensitive to your baby's needs. One study recorded strong brain response in mothers when looking at their own smiling babies versus those who were unfamiliar. That positive ping was also tied to lower anxiety and symptoms of depression, and, scientifically, most resembles falling in love. Which, in a way, it is. Men experience some of the same changes, including a decrease in brain volume when they become fathers. Interestingly, these shifts are more variable but assumed to be tied to the transition to parent.

No matter how much you love your baby, sometimes you'll feel different and conflicting feelings, all at the same time. This ambivalence can be a mix of frustration, anxiety, love, anger, resentment, wonder, and guilt. Though few parents talk about it, feeling this way is entirely normal. There is nothing wrong with you if you find yourself missing the life you had before kids or wonder when (or if) things will ever get easier.

Being a parent is amazing and hard, and every new phase carries its own challenges. Some people who don't enjoy the baby phase love toddlers and vice versa. And it's hard to remember in the moment, but every phase is a season that will pass, usually more quickly than you expect. If you have future children, their seasons will be different. The oft-quoted adage "The days are long, but the years are short" is a helpful refrain when you feel like you're losing it.

Manage your feeds, unfollow anyone who doesn't make you feel good, and remember that the shiny lives you see on social media are not real. Prioritize seeing old friends and make new friends whose kids are similar ages to yours so you can go through it together. You will have your own specific strengths and superpowers as a parent, and it is not useful to compare yourself to anyone else.

GOING BACK TO WORK

Break out the waterproof mascara. For many new parents, the transition back to work feels almost as hard as recovering from birth. If you had the opportunity to spend weeks or months with your baby as the primary caregiver, the idea of leaving them with someone else or in day care can be heartbreaking. Especially since they are only getting more interesting and aware of the world just as you have to do it.

If you read the above and feel guilty that you are looking forward to a life beyond diapers and feedings, that's okay too. Not everyone feels successful in those early months or relishes the newborn phase. Returning to a world that you can control and understand (even while managing a tiny human in the off-hours) can be a confidence boost and help you reconnect with your pre-baby self. There is no right way to feel about this transition, and for a lot of people, it's a mix and changes frequently.

No matter exactly where you are in this moment, here are a few pro tips from career coaches about returning to work after parental leave.

Prepare to go back before you actually go back

Maybe you've been keeping an eye on your inbox throughout your maternity leave. Maybe not. Rather than returning to hundreds or thousands of messages the day you go back to the office, try to get a jump on it and scan for what's most important ahead of time. You can also schedule a quick catch-up with your team or boss before your planned return to see what's changed while you were out.

Plan your first day back in the middle of the week

Rather than diving right into a full workweek, start on a Wednesday, or even a Thursday. The staggered week provides a soft start so you aren't away from your baby five full days in a row.

Ease into it

Keep your schedule as open and flexible as possible. While going back part-time might seem appealing, it means you'll miss meetings and may make it harder to reintegrate with the team.

Talk to your manager and team

This is another do-it-before-you-actually-go-back task that can set the stage for a successful return. Be realistic about your life, your parenting responsibilities, and what you can and cannot do. Make your work hours clear and acknowledge how you will cope with emergencies if they come up. If you plan to work from home more (assuming that's an option), now is a great time to carve out that schedule. This maneuver will help you feel better about what you're committing to do and will help your manager and colleagues to calibrate their expectations (and requests) properly.

Manage expectations about before- and after-hours work

There can be tension between childless coworkers and parents, especially if your job entails responsibilities outside of typical working hours. One example that causes a lot of issues: expecting evening duties to shift entirely to someone without kids (unless they're into it). They have lives too. Hopefully some conversation with your boss happened before you had your baby, but if not, be open about your family's schedule and think about an acceptable compromise that allows time with your baby and to do your job if there is no one else to take things on.

Preview (and plan) your work wardrobe

Even a few months postpartum, you won't look exactly as you did before you were pregnant, and your clothes will not fit the same way. The last thing you'll want to do in the morning when you head back to the office is stress about what to wear. Do a wardrobe audit a few weeks beforehand so you can pull together and plan a few outfits. Store outfits together in your closet or lay out options and take photos to keep in a folder on your phone for easy reference. This is especially useful on the mornings after your baby hasn't slept, and you don't have time to think about it.

Ask for help

Employers want (and are incentivized) to bring back working moms. This means there are an increasing number of workplaces that provide transitional support to make sure you feel confident in your return and can focus on your job rather than worrying about your childcare. As long as it doesn't become the new normal, asking for extra flexibility, assistance, and understanding in those early days is fine.

Be open with your partner

While it may seem most critical that you squeeze in every available moment with your baby before and after work, don't forget about your partner. The transition back to work is a big one for them, too, and involves more responsibility. Keep the lines of communication open, and if you need help—ask. Don't forget to see how they are doing, too. If you're a calendar junkie, throw a meeting on your shared calendar to check in, and make it out for a date night when you can. Printing out a physical version of your family calendar or keeping it on a tablet in the kitchen can help keep everyone on the same page.

Introduce a bottle early

Even if you are exclusively breastfeeding, at some point you will have to pump to keep up supply or let someone else feed the baby during an afternoon or evening out. Getting your baby used to a bottle before you go back to work helps make this transition less difficult. Not to mention, it allows your partner the opportunity to try out feeding, which is a great way for them to bond.

Practice your morning and evening routines

If going back to work is going to meaningfully change your family's schedule, try a few dry runs with your partner. This will reduce stress and prevent some of the shock to your system. It will also help you foresee any scheduling difficulties or hiccups regarding your proposed plan.

Stick to a schedule

If there are certain evenings each week that you know you or your partner will need to work late, set a calendar that allows both of you to have that flexibility without resenting the other. Shared calendars that list childcare information and any other events are one lightweight way to keep track. There are also apps that allow this type of collaboration.

MOM GUILT

Going back to work, or doing anything that doesn't involve your baby, comes with another mental hurdle: mom guilt. Everyone feels shades and different degrees, and it doesn't go away when your baby grows into a toddler or goes to school.

Your baby will change. A lot. Every single day in those early months. They're learning to be a human, after all, which is a long, multistage process that never really ends. Your baby's face, mannerisms, behaviors, sounds, and everything else will evolve as they grow out of the newborn phase and become a more sentient human. It's hard to imagine missing a moment. But unless you plan to never leave your child's side, you will miss something eventually.

Another hard thing: If you utilize childcare, whether it's a nanny or day care, your baby will have other close relationships. There may even be moments when it seems like they prefer that person to you. *Cringe.* But, like pregnancy, raising a child is a marathon, not a sprint. You are stuck with each other for the rest of your lives. The caregiver? Unless it's a close family member, not so much.

It's natural to feel jealous or sad or some combination of a hundred conflicting emotions simultaneously. Already in it? You may already be familiar with several of the following runaway-thought trains. Not there yet? Read and prepare.

I'm going to miss everything!

The idea that you won't witness your baby's first steps because you're at work is enough to reduce many parents to tears. And while that could happen, it's just as likely you'd miss it being in a different room or during a run to the grocery store. There are so many developmental milestones during your baby's life that you cannot possibly catch them all.

My baby is different with me now that I'm back at work.

Your baby will be different as they grow through stages no matter what you do. And letting your baby get to know new people is good for their development. Some babies are timid and shy; others will instantly go to a new person. If your baby is the former, gradual introduction to new adults and other infants is a better way to socialize. But in general, after the first few weeks, exposing them to different people and caretakers helps with long-term growth.

I can't imagine sending my baby to day care or letting someone else take care of them.

This is another tough one if you've had the opportunity to spend time as the primary caregiver. Hopefully, before you gave birth you had time to carefully vet the person who—or place that—will be responsible for your baby. To help with the transition, and to ease your own fears, you may want to take your baby to day care yourself or have the nanny over once or twice before you leave your baby solely in their care. You'll be able to see how the caregiver works, ask any remaining questions, and witness how your baby does in their new environment.

After all that hard work, my milk supply is going to completely dry up.

While it's true that workplaces don't support bring-your-baby-to-work breastfeeding, they are legally required to provide time and space for pumping, which, done regularly, should ensure consistent supply. You can pump right after breastfeeding (an old trick to make your body think you need to make more milk), before you head to work, and as many times as you need to during the day. You'll also need to stick to your guns with scheduling (this is where those prebooked calendar pumping blocks come in handy), because skipping or changing the time you pump will impact your supply. If people try to schedule meetings during those blocks, remind them that pumping is your legal right. Not allowing you to pump means risking clogged ducts, mastitis, and other conditions that could force you to miss work. Worried it's not reflecting well on your ambition? Stay a little later or get a hands-free pumping bra so you can pump while you work.

ALWAYS SOMETHING THERE TO REMIND ME

Now, to a more fun but bizarre topic. Chimeras were monstrous fire-breathing mythological beasts with the body of a lion, the head of a goat on one end, and the head of a snake on the other. The term now describes any fictional being made of disparate parts. Which post-pregnancy is you!

Though it sounds more like science fiction, even though your baby has vacated your uterus, they left something behind: fetal cells. In fact, if you have an older sibling, some of their cells may be all over your body, too, along with your grandmother's and perhaps even your great-grandmother's.

Georg Schmorl first identified fetal microchimerism, or the presence of fetal cells in a mother's body post-birth and published the seminal paper on the topic in 1893. These cells are found everywhere from the brain, lungs, and heart to the thyroid, breast, and skin. Scientists are still working today to understand their purpose. Their presence is thought to reduce the risk of rheumatoid arthritis, certain autoimmune diseases, and breast cancer, and even to improve wound healing. But we don't really know.

This transfer goes both ways. During pregnancy, some of the mom's cells cross the placenta and go into the baby's body, too, and are still found there years later. So really, though your baby is no longer literally in your body, and even after they eventually (hopefully) move out of your house, there is a small part of your child that will never leave.

BIRTH SPACING

This still probably sounds unbelievable, but soon you won't even remember what labor or pregnancy was like.

If you are thinking about your next time around, there are a few things to know about birth spacing. Research indicates the ideal amount of time for your body to fully normalize between pregnancies is eighteen to twenty-four months, especially if you've had a C-section. Sounds like a long time, sure, but it took nine months to get there, and it takes at least that amount of time to find your new normal. If, due to age or circumstance, it isn't possible to wait that long, the downsides of starting sooner are increased odds of preterm birth, low birthweight, and even neonatal morbidity.

The best thing to do: Talk to your doctor about your family goals, see how your body recovers from this pregnancy and birth, and formulate a plan together.

> *I could keep going forever, but I have a publication deadline and two tiny humans that are less tiny every day, so let me leave you with this: Enjoy that newborn smell (someone please figure out how to bottle it)—that scent does not last forever. If you do this again, you'll be too busy chasing the first kid around to fret about every pregnancy symptom and decision. Deep breaths, friend. Speaking of that tiny human, you are not messing everything up. You got this, and you're doing GREAT. Go easy on yourself, and all the other parents out there doing as best they can. We're all in this populating-and-living-on-the-Earth thing together, people. Be kind.*

ACKNOWLEDGMENTS

Toni Morrison wrote: "If there's a book that you want to read, but it hasn't been written yet, then you must write it." That sentiment motivated me to turn my personal journey into this book.

To the readers of *Bumpin*'s first edition who shared their pregnancies, miscarriages, challenges, and questions—thank you for inspiring this revised version.

As with babies, birthing two editions of this book required a lot of help.

To the marvelous Jane van Dis, thanks for sharing your many years of obstetrical expertise and editorial prowess. Your cheerleading and brainstorming and collaboration made it so much better.

To my OG team at Simon and Schuster: Theresa DiMasi, thanks for believing I had this book in me the first time we spoke. Thanks to Kate Davids, Emily Carleton, and Anja Schmidt for helping to bring this book to life. Dondeena Bradley, thank you for doing that magical connection thing you do. For round two, editor extraordinaire Emma Taussig, thank you for joining me for another adventure. Thanks also to the amazing repeat production team of Polly Watson, Nancy Tonik, Laura Levatino, Allison Har-zvi, Jessie McNiel, Ashley Cullina, Liz Casal, Michael Nagin, Jackie Seow, and Patrick Sullivan for all your hard work on both editions.

Many providers and experts sat for interviews on and off the record for this book. Special thanks to Aliza Marogy, ND; Amy Brandon,

MD; Alexandra Brown; Alex Capano, DNP, CRNP, FNP-BC; Carine Carmy; Heather Charmatz; Michaela Cruze; Meleah Ekstrand; Mary Beth Ferrante; Valerie Flaherman, MD; Martina Fogt, MPT; Nara Lee; Myles Lewis; Ronit Menashe; Nina Montgomery; Mercedes Samudio; Sara Stieg; Jackie Stone, MD; Kendra Tolbert, MS, RDN, CDN, LD, RYT, Cert AT; Nina Wilson, CNM, IBCLC; and Danika Wynn, CNM, IBCLC. And thanks to Kalliope White for help facilitating so many great conversations.

Kate Ryder, you and Maven contributed greatly to my personal experience and so many parts of this book—thank you. To the many friends who supported my journey, I am so grateful: Aike Ho, Alyssa Jaffee, Amy Lockwood, Andrew and Nicole Weiss, Anne Devereux-Mills, Arian Van de Carr, Ashlee Adams, Aza Raskin, Chrissy Farr, Christy Habetz, Ciara Devereux, Clare Wylie, Deena Shakir, Jenn Hirsch, Kathy Chan, Kieran Kieckhefer, Kim Lembo, Kim Taylor, Lauren Burns, Linda Avey, Lisa Forster, Megan Miller, Michael Brooks, Morgan Chaney, Ryan Panchardsaram, Scott Gallacher, Stacy Stokes, Suhasini Chandramouli, Susan Coelius Keplinger, and Victoria Graham.

Thanks to my parents, Gayle and Jim Ziegler, for bringing me up to believe that there was nothing I couldn't do, like write this book.

Nick, my hype man and number one cheerleader, you let me bore you with random pregnancy facts, provided the dude's perspective, named this book, helped with edits, kept me going during the rough periods, and, most of all, made me laugh every single day—and still do. I love you so much.

And finally, to my greatest creations, Mr. Baby (a.k.a. TJ) and Dylan: Thank you for making me a mom.

BIBLIOGRAPHY

Preface

Bui, Quoctrung, and Claire Cain Miller. "The Age That Women Have Babies: How a Gap Divides America." *New York Times*. August 4, 2018. https://www.nytimes.com/interactive/2018/08/04/upshot/up-birth-age-gap.html.

California Health Care Foundation. "Improving Maternal Mental Health Care." Accessed November 20, 2023. https://www.chcf.org/project/improving-treatment-of-maternal-mental-health/.

Danielsson, Krissi. "Making Sense of Miscarriage Statistics." Verywell Family. Accessed November 20, 2023. https://www.verywellfamily.com/making-sense-of-miscarriage-statistics-2371721.

Eunice Kennedy Shriver National Institute of Child Health and Human Development. "How Common Is Infertility?" Accessed November 20, 2023. https://www.nichd.nih.gov/health/topics/infertility/conditioninfo/common.

Lyerly, Anne Drapkin, and Ruth R. Faden. "Mothers Matter: Ethics and Research During Pregnancy." *American Medical Association Journal of Ethics* 15, no. 9 (September 2013). https://journalofethics.ama-assn.org/article/mothers-matter-ethics-and-research-during-pregnancy/2013-09.

Martin, Joyce A., et al. "Births: Final Data for 2021." *National Vital Statistics Reports* 72, no. 1 (January 31, 2023). https://www.cdc.gov/nchs/data/nvsr/nvsr72/nvsr72-01.pdf.

Morris, Zoë Slote, et al. "The Answer Is 17 Years, What Is the Question: Understanding Time Lags in Translational Research." *Journal of the Royal Society of Medicine* 104, no. 12 (December 2011): 510–20. https://doi.org/10.1258/jrsm.2011.110180.

World Health Organization. "Infertility Prevalence Estimates, 1990–2021."

April 3, 2023. https://iris.who.int/bitstream/handle/10665/366700 /9789240068315-eng.pdf.

Trimester Zero

Kumar, Naina, and Amit Kant Singh. "Trends of Male Factor Infertility, an Important Cause of Infertility: A Review of Literature." *Journal of Human Reproductive Sciences* 8, no. 4 (2015): 191–96. https://doi .org/10.4103/0974-1208.170370.

Get Ready

American College of Obstetricians and Gynecologists. "Carrier Screening for Genetic Conditions." ACOG Committee Opinion No. 691 (March 2017). https://www.acog.org/-/media/project/acog/acogorg/clinical/files /committee-opinion/articles/2017/03/carrier-screening-for-genetic -conditions.pdf.

Axelsson, Jonatan, et al. "Association Between Paternal Smoking at the Time of Pregnancy and the Semen Quality in Sons." *PLoS ONE* 13, no. 11 (November 2018). https://doi.org/10.1371/journal.pone.0207221.

Baratt, Christopher L. R., et al. "A Global Approach to Addressing the Policy, Research and Social Challenges of Male Reproductive Health." *Human Reproduction Open*, no. 1 (March 21, 2021). https://doi.org /10.1093/hropen/hoab009.

Blanchflower, David G., and Andrew E. Clark. "Children, Unhappiness, and Family Finances: Evidence from One Million Europeans." National Bureau of Economic Research, NBER Working Paper No. 25597, February 2019. https://www.nber.org/papers/w25597.

Blencowe, Hannah, et al. "Folic Acid to Reduce Neonatal Mortality from Neural Tube Disorders." *International Journal of Epidemiology* 39, Supplement 1 (April 2010): i110–21. https://doi.org/10.1093/ije/dyq028.

Care.com. "This Is How Much Child Care Costs in 2023." July 24, 2023. https://www.care.com/c/stories/2423/how-much-does-child-care-cost/.

Catov, Janet M., et al. "Periconceptional Multivitamin Use and Risk of Preterm or Small-for-Gestational-Age Births in the Danish National Birth Cohort." *American Journal of Clinical Nutrition* 94, no. 3 (September 2011): 906–12. https://doi.org/10.3945/ajcn.111.012393.

Centers for Disease Control and Prevention. "Data & Statistics on Birth Defects." Accessed November 20, 2023. https://www.cdc.gov/ncbddd /birthdefects/data.html.

Centers for Disease Control and Prevention. "Folic Acid." Accessed November 20, 2023. https://www.cdc.gov/ncbddd/folicacid/index.html.

Centers for Disease Control and Prevention. "What Is the MTHFR Gene?" Accessed November 20, 2023. https://www.cdc.gov/ncbddd/folicacid /mthfr-gene-and-folic-acid.html.

Chatot, Myriam, et al. "Socioeconomic Differences and the Gender Division of Labor During the Covid-19 Lockdown: Insights from France Using a Mixed Method." *Gender, Work & Organization* 30, no. 4 (July 2023): 1296–316. https://doi.org/10.1111/gwao.12980.

Guo, Liu, et al. "Maternal Iron Supplementation During Pregnancy Affects Placental Function and Iron Status in Offspring." *Journal of Trace Elements in Medicine and Biology* 71 (May 2022). https://doi.org/10.1016/j .jtemb.2022.126950.

Hehemann, Marah C., et al. "Evaluation of the Impact of Marijuana Use on Semen Quality: A Prospective Analysis." *Therapeutic Advances in Urology*, no. 13 (2021). https://doi.org/10.1177/17562872211032484.

Levine, Hagai, et al. "Temporal Trends in Sperm Count: A Systematic Review and MetaRegression Analysis of Samples Collected Globally in the 20th and 21st Centuries." *Human Reproduction Update* 29, no. 2 (March– April 2023): 157–76. https://doi.org/10.1093/humupd/dmac035.

Maven Clinic. "The State of Fertility and Family Benefits in 2023." Accessed November 6, 2023. https://www.mavenclinic.com/interactive -experience/the-state-of-fertility-and-family-benefits-report.

Medscape & CDC. "MTHFR and Birth Defects: Does Type of Folate Matter?" Accessed November 20, 2023. https://www.medscape.com /viewarticle/925368.

Murphy, Susan K., et al. "Cannabinoid Exposure and Altered DNA Methylation in Rat and Human Sperm." *Epigenetics* 13, no. 12 (December 2018): 1208–21. https://doi.org/10.1080/15592294.2018.1554521.

Stroman, Trish, et al. "Why Paid Family Leave Is Good Business." BCG Henderson Institute, February 7, 2017. https://www.bcg.com/publi cations/2017/human-resources-people-organization-why-paid-family -leave-is-good-business.aspx.

US Preventive Forces Task Force. "Folic Acid Supplementation to Prevent Neural Tube Defects." *Journal of the American Medical Association* 330, no. 5 (August 2023): 454–59. https://doi.org/10.1001/jama.2023.12876.

Wald, Nicholas J. "Folic Acid and Neural Tube Defects: Discovery, Debate and the Need for Policy Change." *Journal of Medical Screening* 29, no. 3 (June 23, 2022): 138–46. https://doi.org/10.1177/09691413221 102321.

Wald, Nicholas J. "Postscript to 'Folic Acid and Neural Tube Defects: Discovery, Debate and the Need for Policy Change.'" *Journal of*

Medical Screening 29, no. 3 (2022): 147. https://doi.org/10.1177
/09691413221117464.

Weinhold, Bob. "Epigenetics: The Science of Change." *Environmental Health Perspectives* 114, no. 3 (March 2006): A160–67. https://doi
.org/10.1289/ehp.114-a160.

Wikipedia. "Lucy Wills." Accessed November 20, 2023. https://en.wikipedia
.org/wiki/Lucy_Wills.

Yavorsky, Jill E., et al. "The Production of Inequality: The Gender Division of Labor Across the Transition to Parenthood." *Journal of Marriage and the Family* 77, no. 3 (June 2015): 662–79. https://doi.org/10.1111
/jomf.12189.

Making a Baby

Annan, John Jude Kweku, et al. "Biochemical Pregnancy During Assisted Conception: A Little Bit Pregnant." *Journal of Clinical Medicine Research* 5, no. 4 (August 2013): 269–74. https://doi.org/10.4021/jocmr1008w.

Centers for Disease Control and Prevention. "Birth Data." Last modified September 12, 2023. https://www.cdc.gov/nchs/nvss/births.htm.

Eagleson, Holly. "Your Chances of Getting Pregnant at Every Age." *Parents.* Last modified August 25, 2023. https://www.parents.com/getting
-pregnant/trying-to-conceive/up-your-chances-of-getting-pregnant
-at-every-age/.

Office on Women's Health. "Trying to Conceive." Last updated February 22, 2021. https://www.womenshealth.gov/pregnancy/you-get-pregnant
/trying-conceive.

Steiner, Anne Z., et al. "Association Between Biomarkers of Ovarian Reserve and Infertility Among Older Women of Reproductive Age." *Journal of the American Medical Association* 318, no. 14 (2017): 1367–76. https://
doi.org/10.1001/jama.2017.14588.

Suarez, S. S., and A. A. Pacey. "Sperm Transport in the Female Reproductive Tract." *Human Reproduction Update* 12, no. 1 (January–February 2006): 23–37. https://doi.org/10.1093/humupd/dmi047.

If Things Get Bumpy

Boos, Elise W., et al. "Trends in the Use of Mifepristone for Medical Management of Early Pregnancy Loss From 2016 to 2020." *Journal of the American Medical Association* 330, no. 8 (2023): 766–68. https://
doi.org/10.1001/jama.2023.13628.

Centers for Disease Control and Prevention. "Infertility FAQs." Last updated

April 26, 2023. https://www.cdc.gov/reproductivehealth/infertility/index .htm.

European Society of Human Reproduction and Embryology. "More than 8 Million Babies Born from IVF Since the World's First in 1978." *ScienceDaily*, July 3, 2018. https://www.sciencedaily.com/releases/2018 /07/180703084127.htm.

Kumar, Naina, and Amit Kant Singh. "Trends of Male Factor Infertility, an Important Cause of Infertility: A Review of Literature." *Journal of Human Reproductive Sciences* 8, no. 4 (October–December 2015): 191–96. https://doi.org/10.4103/0974-1208.170370.

Levine, Hagai, et al. "Temporal Trends in Sperm Count: A Systematic Review and Meta-regression Analysis," *Human Reproduction* 23, no. 6 (November–December 2017): 646–59. https://doi.org/10.1093/hum upd/dmx022.

McQueen, Dana B., et al. "Sperm DNA Fragmentation and Recurrent Pregnancy Loss: A Systematic Review and Meta-analysis." *Fertility and Sterility* 112, no. 1 (July 2019): 540–69. https://doi.org/10.1016/j .fertnstert.2019.03.003.

Rossen, Lauren M., et al. "Trends in Risk of Pregnancy Loss Among US Women, 1990–2011." *Paediatric and Perinatal Epidemiology*, no. 1 (January 2018): 19–29. https://doi.org/10.1111/ppe.12417.

Sundermann, Alexandra C., et al. "Alcohol Use in Pregnancy and Miscarriage: A Systematic Review and Meta-analysis." *Alcoholism Clinical and Experimental Research* 43, no. 8 (August 2019): 1606–16. https://doi .org/10.1111/acer.14124.

Wilcox, A. J., et al. "Incidence of Early Loss of Pregnancy." *New England Journal of Medicine* 4, no. 319 (July 1988): 189–94. https://doi.org /10.1056/nejm198807283190401.

The First Trimester

Pregnancy FAQ, Lightning Round

Askling, John, et al. "Sickness in Pregnancy and Sex of Child." *Lancet* 354, no. 9195 (December 11, 1999). https://doi.org/10.1016/S0140 -6736(99)04239-7.

Cook, A. J. C., et al. "Sources of Toxoplasma Infection in Pregnant Women: European Multicentre Case-Control Study." *BMJ* 321, no. 7254 (July 2000): 142–47. https://doi.org/10.1136/bmj.321.7254.142.

Duong, H. T., et al. "Maternal Use of Hot Tub and Major Structural Birth Defects." *Birth Defects Research Part A: Clinical and Molecular*

Teratology 91, no. 9 (September 2011): 836–41. https://doi.org/10.1002/bdra.20831.

Fejzo, M., et al. "GDF15 Linked to Maternal Risk of Nausea and Vomiting During Pregnancy." *Nature* 625, no. 7996 (January 2024): 760–67. https://doi.org/10.1038/s41586-023-06921-9.

Hoekzema, Elseline, et al. "Pregnancy Leads to Long-Lasting Changes in Human Brain Structure." *Nature America* 20, no. 2 (February 2017): 287–96. https://doi.org/10.1038/nn.4458.

Jones, Jeffrey L., et al. "Risk Factors for Toxoplasma Gondii Infection in the United States." *Clinical Infectious Diseases* 49, no. 6 (September 2009): 878–84. https://doi.org/10.1086/605433.

Orchard, Edwina R., et al. "The Maternal Brain Is More Flexible and Responsive at Rest: Effective Connectivity of the Parental Caregiving Network in Postpartum Mothers." *Scientific Reports* 13, no. 4719 (2023). https://doi.org/10.1038/s41598-023-31696-4.

Young, Nicola R., et al. "Does Greater Morning Sickness Predict Carrying a Girl? Analysis of Nausea and Vomiting During Pregnancy from Retrospective Report." *Archives of Gynecology and Obstetrics* 303, no. 5 (2021): 1161–66. https://doi.org/10.1007/s00404-020-05839-1.

Your Care Team Fantasy Draft

American College of Obstetricians and Gynecologists. "Planned Home Births." Committee Opinion No. 697 (April 2017; reaffirmed 2023). https://www.acog.org/clinical/clinical-guidance/committee-opinion/articles/2017/04/planned-home-birth.

Armour, Mike, et al. "Acupuncture and Acupressure for Premenstrual Syndrome." *Cochrane Database of Systematic Reviews*, no. 8, August 14, 2018. https://doi.org/10.1002/14651858.CD005290.pub2.

Bohren, Meghan A., et al. "Continuous Support for Women During Childbirth." *Cochrane Database of Systematic Reviews*, no. 7, July 6, 2017. https://doi.org/10.1002/14651858.CD003766.pub6.

Chicago Lying-In Hospital. "The History of Chicago Lying-In Hospital." Accessed November 20, 2023. https://chicagolyinginboard.uchicago.edu/chicago-lying-in-history/.

Combellick, Joan L., et al. "Midwifery Care During Labor and Birth in the United States." In "Labor Delivery at Term—Part One: Partograms, Labor Disorders, Analgesia/Anesthesia, and Fever," ed. Roberto Romero et al. Supplement, *American Journal of Obstetrics and Gynecology* 228, no. 5 (May 2023): S983-93. https://doi.org/10.1016/j.ajog.2022.09.044.

The Commonwealth Fund. "Maternal Mortality in the United States: A

Primer." December 16, 2020. https://www.commonwealthfund.org/publications/issue-brief-report/2020/dec/maternal-mortality-united-states-primer.

Field, Tiffany. "Pregnancy and Labor Massage." *Expert Review of Obstetrics & Gynecology* 5, no. 2 (January 2014): 177–81. https://doi.org/10.1586/eog.10.12.

Kozhimannil, Katy Backes, et al. "Doula Care, Birth Outcomes, and Costs Among Medicaid Beneficiaries." *American Journal of Public Health* 103, no. 4 (2013): e113–21. https://doi.org/10.2105/AJPH.2012.301201.

Leavitt, Judith W. "Joseph B. DeLee and the Practice of Preventive Obstetrics." *American Journal of Public Health* 78, no. 10 (October 1988): 1353–60. https://ajph.aphapublications.org/doi/pdf/10.2105/AJPH.78.10.1353.

Liddle, S. D., and V. Pennick. "Interventions for Preventing and Treating Low-Back and Pelvic Pain During Pregnancy." *Cochrane Database of Systematic Reviews*, no. 9, September 30, 2015. https://doi.org/10.1002/14651858.CD001139.pub4.

Niles, P. Mimi, et al. "Examining Respect, Autonomy, and Mistreatment in Childbirth in the US: Do Provider Type and Place of Birth Matter?" *Reproductive Health*, no. 20 (May 2023): 67. https://doi.org/10.1186/s12978-023-01584-1.

Scientific American. "The US Needs More Midwives for Better Maternity Care." February 1, 2019. https://www.scientificamerican.com/article/the-u-s-needs-more-midwives-for-better-maternity-care/.

Smith, Caroline A., et al. "Acupuncture or Acupressure for Pain Management During Labour." *Cochrane Database of Systematic Reviews*, no. 2, February 7, 2020. https://doi.org/10.1002/14651858.CD009232.pub2.

Wertz, Richard W., et al. *Lying-In: A History of Childbirth in America.* New Haven: Yale University Press, 1989.

Things to Avoid

American Cancer Society. "Marijuana and Cancer." Accessed November 20, 2023. https://www.cancer.org/treatment/treatments-and-side-effects/complementary-and-alternative-medicine/marijuana-and-cancer.html.

American College of Obstetricians and Gynecologists. "Tobacco, Alcohol, Drugs, and Pregnancy." Accessed November 20, 2023. https://www.acog.org/womens-health/faqs/tobacco-alcohol-drugs-and-pregnancy.

Anderson, Tatiana M., et al. "Maternal Smoking Before and During Pregnancy and the Risk of Sudden Unexpected Infant Death." *Pediatrics* 143, no. 4 (April 2019). https://doi.org/10.1542/peds.2018-3325.

Bonn-Miller, Marcel O., et al. "Labeling Accuracy of Cannabidiol Extracts Sold Online." *Journal of the American Medical Association* 318, no. 17 (November 2017): 1708–9. https://doi.org/10.1001/jama.2017.11909.

Centers for Disease Control and Prevention. "Substance Use During Pregnancy." Accessed November 20, 2023. https://www.cdc.gov/repro ductivehealth/maternalinfanthealth/substance-abuse/substance-abuse -during-pregnancy.htm.

Conover, Wayne B., et al. "Maternal Cardiovascular Response to Caffeine Infusion in the Pregnant Ewe." *American Journal of Obstetrics & Gynecology* 145, no. 5 (March 1983): 534–38. https://doi.org/10.1016/0002 -9378(83)91191-2.

Genetic Alliance; District of Columbia Department of Health. "Appendix D: Teratogens/Prenatal Substance Abuse." In *Understanding Genetics: A District of Columbia Guide for Patients and Health Professionals.* Washington, DC: Genetic Alliance, 2010. https://www.ncbi.nlm.nih .gov/books/NBK132140/.

Griffiths, Sarah K., and Jeremy P. Campbell. "Placental Structure, Function and Drug Transfer." *Continuing Education in Anaesthesia Critical Care & Pain* 15, no. 2 (April 2015): 84–89. https://doi.org/10.1093 /bjaceaccp/mku013.

Gunn, J. K., et al. "Prenatal Exposure to Cannabis and Maternal and Child Health Outcomes: A Systematic Review and Meta-analysis." *BMJ Open* 6, no. 4 (April 2016). https://doi.org/10.1136/bmjopen-2015-009986.

Hammer, Raphaël, and Elise Rapp. "Women's Views and Experiences of Occasional Alcohol Consumption During Pregnancy: A Systematic Review of Qualitative Studies and Their Recommendations." *Midwifery* 111 (August 2022). https://doi.org/10.1016/j.midw.2022.103 357.

May, P. A., et al. "Prevalence of Fetal Alcohol Spectrum Disorders in 4 US Communities." *Journal of the American Medical Association* 319, no. 5 (February 2018): 474–82. https://doi.org/10.1001/jama.2017.21896.

Murphy, Susan K., et al. "Cannabinoid Exposure and Altered DNA Methylation in Rat and Human Sperm." *Epigenetics* 13, no. 12 (December 2018): 1208–21. https://doi.org/10.1080/15592294.2018.1 554521.

Trivedi, M. K., et al. "A Review of the Safety of Cosmetic Procedures During Pregnancy and Lactation." *International Journal of Women's Dermatology* 3, no. 1 (February 2017): 6–10. https://doi.org/10.1016/j .ijwd.2017.01.005.

Pregnant Bodies Are Strong Bodies

American College of Obstetricians and Gynecologists. "Weight Gain During Pregnancy." Committee Opinion No. 548 (Reaffirmed 2023). https://www.acog.org/Clinical-Guidance-and-Publications/Committee-Opinions/Committee-on-Obstetric-Practice/Weight-Gain-During-Pregnancy.

Bahls, Martin, et al. "Mothers' Exercise During Pregnancy Programmes Vasomotor Function in Adult Offspring." *Experimental Physiology* 99, no. 1 (January 2014): 205–19. https://doi.org/10.1113/expphysiol.2013.075978.

Cooper, Danielle B., and Lily Yang. *Pregnancy and Exercise*. Treasure Island, FL: StatPearls Publishing, 2023. https://www.ncbi.nlm.nih.gov/books/NBK430821/.

Labonte-Lemoyne, Elise, et al. "Exercise During Pregnancy Enhances Cerebral Maturation in the Newborn: A Randomized Controlled Trial." *Journal of Clinical and Experimental Neuropsychology* 39, no. 4 (2017): 347–54. https://doi.org/10.1080/13803395.2016.1227427.

To Test or Not to Test?

American Diabetes Association Professional Practice Committee. "Management of Diabetes in Pregnancy: Standards of Care in Diabetes—2024." *Diabetes Care* 47 (January 2024), Supplement 1: S282–S294. https://doi.org/10.2337/dc24-S015.

Brambati, B., and G. Simoni. "Diagnosis of Fetal Trisomy 21 in First Trimester." *Lancet* 321, no. 8324 (March 12, 1983): 586. https://doi.org/10.1016/S0140-6736(83)92831-3.

Centers for Disease Control and Prevention. "Gestational Diabetes." Accessed November 20, 2023. https://www.cdc.gov/diabetes/basics/gestational.html.

Centers for Disease Control and Prevention. "Group B Strep." Accessed November 20, 2023. https://www.cdc.gov/groupbstrep/.

Hartwig, Tanja Schlaikjær, et al. "Cell-Free Fetal DNA for Genetic Evaluation in Copenhagen Pregnancy Loss Study: A Prospective Cohort Study." *Lancet* 401, no. 10378 (March 4, 2023): 762–71. https://doi.org/10.1016/S0140-6736(22)02610-1.

Mayo Clinic. "Amniocentesis." Accessed November 20, 2023. https://www.mayoclinic.org/tests-procedures/amniocentesis/about/pac-20392914.

Mayo Clinic. "First Trimester Screening." Last modified August 26, 2022. https://www.mayoclinic.org/tests-procedures/first-trimester-screening/about/pac-20394169.

Mayo Clinic. "Rh Factor Blood Test." Accessed November 20, 2023. https://www.mayoclinic.org/tests-procedures/rh-factor/about/pac-20394960.

Nagase, Hiromi, et al. "Fetal Outcome of Trisomy 18 Diagnosed After 22 Weeks of Gestation: Experience of 123 Cases at a Single Perinatal Center." *Congenital Abnormalities* 56, no. 1 (January 2016): 35–40. https://doi.org/10.1111/cga.12118.

Nicolson, Malcolm, and John E. E. Fleming. *Imaging and Imagining the Fetus: The Development of Obstetric Ultrasound.* Baltimore: Johns Hopkins University Press, 2013. https://muse.jhu.edu/.

US Food & Drug Administration. "Ultrasound Imaging." Last modified September 28, 2020. https://www.fda.gov/radiation-emitting-products/medical-imaging/ultrasound-imaging.

The Second Trimester
What Do I Actually Need to Buy?

Lee, Helena. "Why Finnish Babies Sleep in Cardboard Boxes." *BBC News*, June 4, 2013. https://www.bbc.com/news/magazine-22751415.

Terveyden Ja Hyvinvoinnin Laitos. "Finland's Low Infant Mortality Has Multiple Contributing Factors." January 27, 2017. https://blogi.thl.fi/finlands-low-infant-mortality-has-multiple-contributing-factors/.

Meet Your Pelvic Floor

Beckmann, M. M., and O. M. Stock. "Antenatal Perineal Massage for Reducing Perineal Trauma." *Cochrane Database of Systematic Reviews*, no. 4, April 30, 2013. https://doi.org/10.1002/14651858.CD005123.pub3.

Benvenuti, F., et al. "Reeducative Treatment of Female Genuine Stress Incontinence." *American Journal of Physical Medicine* 66, no. 4 (August 1987): 155–68. https://www.ncbi.nlm.nih.gov/pubmed/3674220.

Du, Y., et al. "The Effect of Antenatal Pelvic Floor Muscle Training on Labor and Delivery Outcomes: A Systematic Review with Meta-analysis." *International Urogynecology Journal* 26, no. 10 (October 2015): 1415–27. https://doi.org/10.1007/s00192-015-2654-4.

Keller, Jessica, et al. "Diastasis Recti Abdominis: A Survey of Women's Health Specialists for Current Physical Therapy Clinical Practice for Postpartum Women." *Journal of Women's Health Physical Therapy* 36, no. 3 (September–December 2012): 131–42. https://doi.org/10.1097/JWH.0b013e318276f35f.

Radzimińska, Agnieszka, et al. "The Impact of Pelvic Floor Muscle Training on the Quality of Life of Women with Urinary Incontinence. A Systematic Literature Review." *Clinical Interventions in Aging* 13 (2018): 957–65. https://doi.org/10.2147/CIA.S160057.

Sperstad, J. B., et al. "Diastasis Recti Abdominis During Pregnancy and 12 Months After Childbirth: Prevalence, Risk Factors and Report of Lumbopelvic Pain." *British Journal of Sports Medicine* 50, no. 17 (September 2016): 1092–96. https://bjsm.bmj.com/content/50/17/1092.

Woodley, S. J., et al. "Pelvic Floor Muscle Training for Prevention and Treatment of Urinary and Faecal Incontinence in Antenatal and Postnatal Women." *Cochrane Database of Systematic Reviews*, no. 12, December 22, 2017. https://doi.org/10.1002/14651858.CD007471.pub3.

It's Not a Birth *Plan*—It's Preferences

American College of Nurse-Midwives. "Delayed Umbilical Cord Clamping Position Statement." May 2014. http://www.midwife.org/ACNM/files /ACNMLibraryData/UPLOADFILENAME/000000000290/Delayed -Umbilical-Cord-Clamping-May-2014.pdf.

American College of Obstetricians and Gynecologists. "Cord Blood Banking." July 2022. https://www.acog.org/womens-health/faqs/cord-blood-banking.

Borup, Lissa, et al. "Acupuncture as Pain Relief During Delivery: A Randomized Controlled Trial." *Birth* 36, no. 1 (March 2009): 5–12. https://doi.org/10.1111/j.1523-536X.2008.00290.x.

Buser, G. L., et al. "Notes from the Field: Late-Onset Infant Group B Streptococcus Infection Associated with Maternal Consumption of Capsules Containing Dehydrated Placenta—Oregon." *Morbidity and Mortality Weekly Report* 66, no. 25 (June 30, 2017): 677–78. http:// dx.doi.org/10.15585/mmwr.mm6625a5.

Cepeda-Emiliani, A., et al. "Immunohistological Study of the Density and Distribution of Human Penile Neural Tissue: Gradient Hypothesis." *International Journal of Impotence Research* 35 (2023): 286–305. https://doi.org/10.1038/s41443-022-00561-9.

Cho, Eun Hee, et al. "The Effects of Aromatherapy on Intensive Care Unit Patients' Stress and Sleep Quality: A Nonrandomised Controlled Trial." *Evidence-Based Complementary and Alternative Medicine* (December 2017). https://doi.org/10.1155/2017/2856592.

Cluett, E. R., and A. Cuthbert. "Immersion in Water During Labour and Birth." *Cochrane Database of Systematic Reviews*, no. 5, May 16, 2018. https://doi.org/10.1002/14651858.CD000111.pub4.

Cochrane Complementary Medicine. "The Effect of TENS for Pain Relief in Labor." Accessed June 22, 2019. https://cam.cochrane.org /effect-tens-pain-relief-labor.

Collier, Roger. "Circumcision Indecision: The Ongoing Saga of the World's Most Popular Surgery." *Canadian Medical Association Journal* 183, no. 17 (November 2011): 1961–62. https://doi.org/10.1503/cmaj.109 -4021.

Downe, S., et al. "Self-Hypnosis for Intrapartum Pain Management in Pregnant Nulliparous Women: A Randomised Controlled Trial of Clinical Effectiveness." *BJOG* 122, no. 9 (August 2015): 1226–34. https://doi.org/10.1111/1471-0528.13433.

Farr, Alex, et al. "Human Placentophagy: A Review." *American Journal of Obstetrics and Gynecology* 218, no. 4 (April 2018): 401.E1–11. https:// doi.org/10.1016/j.ajog.2017.08.016.

French, Cynthia A., et al. "Labor Epidural Analgesia and Breastfeeding: A Systematic Review." *Journal of Human Lactation* 32, no. 3 (August 2016): 507–20. https://doi.org/10.1177/0890334415623779.

Green, Josephine M., and Helen A. Baston. "Feeling in Control During Labor: Concepts, Correlates, and Consequences." *Birth* 30, no. 4 (January 2004): 235–47. https://doi.org/10.1046/j.1523-536X.2003.00253.x.

Gryder, L. K., et al. "Effects of Human Maternal Placentophagy on Maternal Postpartum Iron Status: A Randomized, Double-Blind, Placebo-Controlled Pilot Study." *Journal of Midwifery & Women's Health* 62, no. 1 (January 2017): 68–79. https://doi.org/10.1111/jmwh.12549.

Hart-Cooper, Geoffrey D., et al. "Circumcision of Privately Insured Males Aged 0 to 18 Years in the United States." *Pediatrics* 134, no. 5 (November 2014): 950–56. https://doi.org/10.1542/peds.2014-1007.

Hitzeman, Nathan, and Shannon Chin. "Epidural Analgesia for Labor Pain." *American Family Physician* 86, no. 3 (August 2012): 241–42. https:// www.aafp.org/afp/2012/0801/p241.html.

Jaafar, S. H., et al. "Rooming-In for New Mother and Infant Versus Separate Care for Increasing the Duration of Breastfeeding." *Cochrane Database of Systematic Reviews*, no. 8, August 26, 2016. https://doi.org/10 .1002/14651858.CD006641.pub3.

Katheria, Anup C., et al. "Umbilical Cord Milking Versus Delayed Cord Clamping in Preterm Infants." *Pediatrics* 136, no. 1 (July 2015): 61–69. https://doi.org/10.1542/peds.2015-0368.

Krieger, John N., et al. "Adult Male Circumcision: Effects on Sexual Function and Sexual Satisfaction in Kisumu, Kenya." *Journal of Sexual Medicine* 5, no. 11 (November 2008): 2610–22. https://doi .org/10.1111/j.1743-6109.2008.00979.x.

Loewenberg-Weisband, Yiska, et al. "Epidural Analgesia and Severe Perineal Tears: A Literature Review and Large Cohort Study." *Journal of*

Maternal-Fetal & Neonatal Medicine 27, no. 18 (March 2014): 1864–69. https://www.doi.org/10.3109/14767058.2014.889113.

McDonal, S. J. "Effect of Timing of Umbilical Cord Clamping of Term Infants on Maternal and Neonatal Outcomes." *Cochrane Database of Systematic Reviews*, no. 7, July 11, 2013. https://doi.org/10.1002/14651858.CD004074.pub3.

Morris, Brian J., et al. "Does Male Circumcision Affect Sexual Function, Sensitivity, or Satisfaction?—A Systematic Review." *Journal of Sexual Medicine* 10, no. 11 (August 2013): 2644–57. https://www.jsm.jsexmed.org/article/S1743-6095(15)30172-7/.

Moscucci, O. "Holistic Obstetrics: The Origins of 'Natural Childbirth' in Britain." *Postgraduate Medical Journal* 79, no. 929 (March 2003): 168–73. https://doi.org/10.1136/pmj.79.929.168.

Osterman, Michelle J. K., and Joyce A. Martin. "Epidural and Spinal Anesthesia Use During Labor: 27-State Reporting Area, 2008." *National Vital Statistics Reports* 59, no. 5 (April 6, 2011). https://www.cdc.gov/nchs/data/nvsr/nvsr59/nvsr59_05.pdf.

Ramsay, Michael A. E. "John Snow, MD: Anaesthetist to the Queen of England and Pioneer Epidemiologist." *Baylor University Medical Center Proceedings* 19, no. 1 (2006): 24–28. https://doi.org/10.1080/08998280.2006.11928120.

Reynolds, Juli, et al. "Using Aromatherapy in the Clinical Setting: Making Sense of Scents." *American Nurse Today* 13, no. 6 (June 2018). https://www.americannursetoday.com/aromatherapy-clinical-setting/.

Smith, C. A., et al. "Massage, Reflexology and Other Manual Methods for Pain Management in Labour." *Cochrane Database of Systematic Reviews*, no. 3, March 28, 2018. https://doi.org/10.1002/14651858.CD009290.pub3.

Sundermann, Alexandra C., et al. "Alcohol Use in Pregnancy and Miscarriage: A Systematic Review and Meta-analysis." *Alcoholism Clinical & Experimental Research* 43, no. 8 (August 2019): 1606–16. https://doi.org/10.1111/acer.14124.

Weiss, Helen A., et al. "Complications of Circumcision in Male Neonates, Infants and Children: A Systematic Review." *BMC Urology* 10, no. 2 (February 2010). https://doi.org/10.1186/1471-2490-10-2.

Young, Sharon M., et al. "Ingestion of Steamed and Dehydrated Placenta Capsules Does Not Affect Postpartum Plasma Prolactin Levels or Neonatal Weight Gain: Results from a Randomized, Double-Bind, Placebo-Controlled Pilot Study." *Journal of Midwifery & Women's Health* 64, no. 4 (July–August 2019): 443–50. https://doi.org/10.1111/jmwh.12955.

The Third Trimester
Life Right Before—and After—Birth

Modi, Rohan, et al. "Implementation of a Defecation Posture Modification Device: Impact on Bowel Movement Patterns in Healthy Subjects." *Journal of Clinical Gastroenterology* 53, no. 3 (March 2019): 216–19. https://doi.org/10.1097/MCG.0000000000001143.

Pew Research Center. "Almost 1 in 5 Stay-at-Home Parents in the US Are Dads." Accessed November 20, 2023. https://www.pewresearch.org/short -reads/2023/08/03-almost-1-in-5-stay-at-home-parents-in-the-us-are-dads.

The Big Event

Al-Kuran, O., et al. "The Effect of Late Pregnancy Consumption of Date Fruit on Labour and Delivery." *Journal of Obstetrics and Gynaecology* 31, no. 1 (January 2011): 29–31. https://doi.org/10.3109/01443615.2010.522267.

American Academy of Pediatrics. "Newborn Hearing Screening FAQs." Accessed November 20, 2023. https://www.healthychildren.org/English /ages-stages/baby/Pages/Purpose-of-Newborn-Hearing-Screening.aspx.

American College of Obstetricians and Gynecologists. "Delayed Umbilical Cord Clamping After Birth." Reaffirmed 2023. https://www.acog.org /clinical/clinical-guidance/committee-opinion/articles/2020/12/de layed-umbilical-cord-clamping-after-birth.

American College of Obstetricians and Gynecologists. "If Your Baby Is Breech." Last modified August 2022. https://www.acog.org/womens -health/faqs/if-your-baby-is-breech.

Athile, Yoann, et al. "Association Between Hospitals' Caesarean Delivery Rates for Breech Presentation and Their Success Rates for External Cephalic Version." *European Journal of Obstetrics & Gynecology* 270 (March 2022): 156–63. https://doi.org/10.1016/j.ejogrb.2022.01.007.

Bhatia, Manjeet Singh, and Anurag Jhanjee. "Tokophobia: A Dread of Pregnancy." *Industrial Psychiatry Journal* 21, no. 2 (July–December 2012): 158–59. https://doi.org/10.4103/0972-6748.119649.

Caughey, Aaron B., et al. *Maternal and Neonatal Outcomes of Elective Induction of Labor.* Rockville, MD: Agency for Healthcare Research and Quality, 2009. https://www.ncbi.nlm.nih.gov/books/NBK38683/.

Centers for Disease Control and Prevention. "Critical Congenital Heart Defects." Accessed November 20, 2023. https://www.cdc.gov/ncbddd /heartdefects/cchd-facts.html.

Dahlen, H. G., et al. "Perineal Outcomes and Maternal Comfort Related to the Application of Perineal Warm Packs in the Second Stage of Labor:

A Randomized Controlled Trial." *Birth* 34, no. 4 (December 2007): 282–90. https://doi.org/10.1111/j.1523-536X.2007.00186.x.

Grobman, William A., et al. "Labor Induction Versus Expectant Management in Low-Risk Nulliparous Women." *New England Journal of Medicine*, no. 379 (August 2018): 513–23. https://doi.org/10.1056/NEJ Moa1800566.

Hakem, Emmanuel, et al. "External Cephalic Version: A 10-year Review of Practice," *European Journal of Obstetrics & Gynecology* 258 (March 2021): 414–17. https://doi.org/10.1016/j.ejogrb.2021.01.044.

Hannah, Mary E. "Planned Elective Cesarean Section: A Reasonable Choice for Some Women?" *Canadian Medical Association Journal* 170, no. 5 (March 2, 2004): 813–14. https://doi.org/10.1503/cmaj.1032002.

Harper, Terry C., et al. "A Randomized Controlled Trial of Acupuncture for Initiation of Labor in Nulliparous Women." *Journal of Maternal-Fetal & Neonatal Medicine* 19, no. 8 (2006): 465–70. https://doi.org /10.1080/14767050600730740.

Hersh, Alyssa R., et al. "Analysis of Obstetric Outcomes by Hospital Location, Volume, and Teaching Status Associated with Non-medically Indicated Induction of Labor at 39 Weeks." *Journal of the American Medical Association Network Open* 6, no. 4 (2023). https://doi.org/10.1001 /jamanetworkopen.2023.9167.

Jakobsson, H. E., et al. "Decreased Gut Microbiota Diversity, Delayed Bacteroidetes Colonisation and Reduced Th1 Responses in Infants Delivered by Caesarean Section." *Gut* 62, no. 4 (April 2014): 559–66. https://doi.org/10.1136/gutjnl-2012-303249.

Khambalia, Amina Z., et al. "Predicting Date of Birth and Examining the Best Time to Date a Pregnancy." *International Journal of Gynecology & Obstetrics* 123, no. 2 (November 2013): 105–9. https://doi.org /10.1016/j.ijgo.2013.05.007.

Labor, Simona, and Simon Maguire. "The Pain of Labour." *British Journal of Pain* 2, no. 2 (December 2, 2008). https://doi.org/10.1177 /204946370800200205.

Liu, Shiliang, et al. "Maternal Mortality and Severe Morbidity Associated with Low-Risk Planned Cesarean Delivery Versus Planned Vaginal Delivery at Term." *Canadian Medical Association Journal* 176, no. 4 (February 13, 2007): 455–60. https://doi.org/10.1503/cmaj.060870.

Mayo Clinic. "Labor Induction." Accessed November 20, 2023. https://www .mayoclinic.org/tests-procedures/labor-induction/about/pac-20385141.

Oberg, Anna S., et al. "Maternal and Fetal Genetic Contributions to Postterm Birth: Familial Clustering in a Population-Based Sample of 475,429

Swedish Births." *American Journal of Epidemiology* 177, no. 6 (March 15, 2013): 531–37. https://doi.org/10.1093/aje/kws244.

Palacio, Montse, et al. "Meta-analysis of Studies on Biochemical Marker Tests for the Diagnosis of Premature Rupture of Membranes: Comparison of Performance Indexes." *BMC Pregnancy and Childbirth* 14, no. 183 (May 2014). https://doi.org/10.1186/1471-2393-14-183.

Razali, Nuguelis, et al. "Date Fruit Consumption at Term: Effect on Length of Gestation, Labour and Delivery." *Journal of Obstetrics and Gynaecology* 37, no. 5 (July 2017): 595–600. https://doi.org/10.1080/0 1443615.2017.1283304.

Rortveit, Guri, et al. "Urinary Incontinence After Vaginal Delivery or Cesarean Section." *New England Journal of Medicine*, no. 348 (March 6, 2003): 900–907. https://doi.org/10.1056/NEJMoa021788.

Smith, Caroline A., M. Armour, and H. G. Dahle. "Acupuncture or Acupressure for Induction of Labour." *Cochrane Database of Systematic Reviews*, no. 10, October 17, 2017. https://doi.org/10.1002/14651 858.CD002962.pub4.

Smith, Gordon C. S. "Use of Time to Event Analysis to Estimate the Normal Duration of Human Pregnancy." *Human Reproduction* 16, no. 7 (July 2001): 1497–500. https://doi.org/10.1093/humrep/16.7.1497.

Smith, M., et al. "External Cephalic Version in Cases of Breech Presentation: Renaissance of a Well-Known Procedure?" *Gynecological Obstetric Review* 49, no. 1 (2009): 29–34. https://doi.org/10.1159/000184443.

The Fourth Trimester

Deussen, A. R., et al. "Analgesia for Relief of Pains Due to Uterine Cramping/ Involution After Birth." *Cochrane Database of Systematic Reviews*, no. 5, May 11, 2011. https://doi.org/10.1002/14651858.CD004908.pub2.

O'Brien, A. P., et al. "New Fathers' Perinatal Depression and Anxiety-Treatment Options: An Integrative Review." *American Journal of Men's Health* 11, no. 4 (July 2017): 863–76. https://doi.org/10.1177 /1557988316669047.

Recovery

American College of Obstetricians and Gynecologists. "Optimizing Postpartum Care." Committee Opinion No. 736 (May 2017; reaffirmed 2021). https://www.acog.org/clinical/clinical-guidance/committee-opinion /articles/2018/05/optimizing-postpartum-care.

Cheifetz, Oren S., et al. "The Effect of Abdominal Support on Functional Outcomes in Patients Following Major Abdominal Surgery: A Randomized Controlled Trial." *Physiotherapy Canada* 62, no. 3 (Summer 2010): 242–53. https://doi.org/10.3138/physio.62.3.242.

Garbarino, Abigail H., et al. "Current Trends in Psychiatric Education Among Obstetrics and Gynecology Residency Programs." *Academic Psychiatry* 43, no. 3 (June 2019): 294–99. https://doi.org/10.1007/s40596-019-01 018-w.

Keeler, Jessica, et al. "Diastasis Recti Abdominis: A Survey of Women's Health Specialists for Current Physical Therapy Clinical Practice for Postpartum Women." *Journal of Women's Health Physical Therapy* 36, no. 3 (September–December 2012): 131–42. https://doi.org/10.1097 /JWH.0b013e318276f35f.

O'Connor, Elizabeth, et al. "Interventions to Prevent Perinatal Depression: Evidence Report and Systematic Review for the US Preventive Services Task Force." *Journal of the American Medical Association* 321, no. 6 (2019): 588–601. https://doi.org/10.1001/jama.2018.20865.

Woolner, Andrea Mary, et al. "The Impact of Third- or Fourth-Degree Perineal Tears on the Second Pregnancy: A Cohort Study of 182,445 Scottish Women." *PLoS ONE*, April 11, 2019. https://doi.org/10.1371 /journal.pone.0215180.

Feeding Time

Centers for Disease Control and Prevention. "Breastfeeding Is an Investment in Health, Not Just a Lifestyle Decision." Accessed November 20, 2023. https://www.cdc.gov/breastfeeding/about-breastfeeding/why-it-matters .html.

Centers for Disease Control and Prevention. "Breastfeeding Report Card, United States 2022." Last reviewed August 21, 2022. https://www.cdc .gov/breastfeeding/data/reportcard.htm.

Der, Geoff, G. David Batty, and Ian J. Deary. "Results from the PROBIT Breastfeeding Trial May Have Been Overinterpreted." *Archives of General Psychiatry* 65, no. 12 (2008): 1456–57. http://doi.org/10.1001 /archpsyc.65.12.1456-b.

Der, Geoff, et al. "Effect of Breast Feeding on Intelligence in Children: Prospective Study, Sibling Pairs Analysis and Meta-analysis." *BMJ* 333, no. 945 (August 2006). https://doi.org/10.1136/bmj.38978.699583.55.

Eidelman, Arthur I., et al. "Breastfeeding and the Use of Human Milk." *Pediatrics* 129, no. 3 (2012). https://pediatrics.aappublications.org /content/129/3/e827.

Flaherman, Valerie J., et al. "Effect of Early Limited Formula on Breastfeeding Duration in the First Year of Life: A Randomized Clinical Trial." *Journal of the American Medical Association Pediatrics* 173, no. 8 (2019): 729–35. https://www.doi.org/10.1001/jamapediatrics.2019.1424.

Flaherman, Valerie, et al. "Health Care Utilization in the First Month After Birth and Its Relationship to Newborn Weight Loss and Method of Feeding." *Academic Pediatrics* 18, no. 6 (August 2018): 677–84. https://doi.org/10.1016/j.acap.2017.11.005.

Grand View Research. "Breastfeeding Accessories Market Size, Share & Trends Analysis Report by Product (Nipple Care Products, Breast Shells, Breast Pads, Breastmilk Storage & Feeding), by Region, and Segment Forecasts, 2023–2030." 2023. https://www.grandview research.com/industry-analysis/breastfeeding-accessories-market.

Institute of Medicine (US) Committee on Nutritional Status During Pregnancy and Lactation. "Who Breastfeeds in the United States?" In *Nutrition During Lactation.* Washington, DC: National Academies Press, 1991. https://www.ncbi.nlm.nih.gov/books/NBK235588/.

Keim, Sarah A., et al. "Cow's Milk Contamination of Human Milk Purchased Via the Internet." *Pediatrics* 135, no. 5 (May 2015): e1157–62. https://doi.org/10.1542/peds.2014-3554.

Kramer, M. S., et al. "Promotion of Breastfeeding Intervention Trial (PROBIT): A Randomized Trial in the Republic of Belarus." *Journal of the American Medical Association* 285, no. 4 (January 2001): 413–20. http://doi.org/10.1001/jama.285.4.413.

Kramer, Michael S., et al. "Breastfeeding and Child Cognitive Development: New Evidence from a Large Randomized Trial." *Archives of General Psychiatry* 65, no. 5 (2008): 578–84. https://doi.org/10.1001/archpsyc.65.5.578.

Muller, Mike. "The Baby Killer." *War on Want*, March 1974. Available at http://archive.babymilkaction.org/pdfs/babykiller.pdf.

Papastavrou, M., et al. "Breastfeeding in the Course of History." *Journal of Pediatrics and Neonatal Care* 2, no. 6 (September 2015). http://doi.org/10.15406/jpnc.2015.02.00096.

Petherick, Anna. "Holder Pasteurization Has Limited Impact on the Nutrients in Human Milk." *Splash! Milk Science Update*, August 2017. https://milkgenomics.org/article/holder-pasteurization-limited-impact-nutrients-human-milk/.

Ryan, Rachel A., et al. "Use of Galactagogues to Increase Milk Production Among Breastfeeding Mothers in the United States: A Descriptive Study." *Journal of the Academy of Nutrition and Dietetics*, May 24, 2023. https://doi.org/10.1016/j.jand.2023.05.019.

Stevens, Emily E., Thelma E. Patrick, and Rita Pickler. "A History of Infant Feeding." *Journal of Perinatal Education* 18, no. 2 (Spring 2009): 32–39. http://doi.org/10.1624/105812409X426314.

Tuttle, Cynthia Reeves, and Wendy I. Slavitt. "Establishing the Business Case for Breastfeeding." *Breastfeeding Medicine* 4, Supplement 1 (October 2009). https://doi.org/10.1089/bfm.2009.0031.

US Bureau of Labor Statistics. "Employee Benefits Survey." Accessed November 20, 2023. https://www.bls.gov/ncs/ebs/benefits/2014/owner ship/civilian/table32a.htm.

Ventura, K. "Does Breastfeeding Shape Food Preferences? Links to Obesity." *Annals of Nutrition & Metabolism* 70, no. 3 (2017): 8–15. https://doi .org/10.1159/000478757.

World Health Organization. "The Physiological Basis of Breastfeeding." In *Infant and Young Child Feeding: Model Chapter for Textbooks for Medical Students and Allied Health Professionals*. Geneva: World Health Organization, 2009. https://www.ncbi.nlm.nih.gov/books/NBK 148970/.

Your New Roommate

Wilkinson, Carol L., et al. "Quantitative Evaluation of Content and Age Concordance Across Developmental Milestone Checklists." *Journal of Developmental and Behavioral Pediatrics*, June 4, 2019. https://doi .org/10.1097/DBP.0000000000000695.

Wong, Kate. "Why Humans Give Birth to Helpless Babies." *Scientific American*, August 28, 2012. https://blogs.scientificamerican.com /observations/why-humans-give-birth-to-helpless-babies/.

Transitions

Barrett, Jennifer, et al. "Maternal Affect and Quality of Parenting Experiences Are Related to Amygdala Response to Infant Faces." *Social Neuroscience* 7, no. 3 (2012): 252–68, https://doi.org/10.1080 /17470919.2011.609907.

Boddy, Amy M., et al. "Fetal Microchimerism and Maternal Health: A Review and Evolutionary Analysis of Cooperation and Conflict Beyond the Womb." *BioEssays* 37, no. 10 (October 2015): 1106–18. https://doi .org/10.1002/bies.201500059.

Lapaire, O., et al. "Georg Schmorl on Trophoblasts in the Maternal Circulation." *Placenta* 28, no. 1 (January 2007): 1–5. https://doi.org/10 .1016/j.placenta.2006.02.004.

Verneris, Michael. "Fetal Microchimerism—What Our Children Leave Behind." *Blood* 102, no. 10 (2003): 3465–66. https://doi.org/10.1182/blood-2003-09-3027.

Wikipedia. "Microchimerism." Accessed November 20, 2023. https://en.wikipedia.org/wiki/Microchimerism.

INDEX

Note: Page references in italics indicate illustrations, and a t *indicates a table.*

AAP (American Academy of
   Pediatrics), 327–28
abortion (termination of a
   pregnancy), 37–38, 145
acetaminophen, 270
acid reflux, 58–59, 111, 114
acne, 60, 106–8t
acupuncture
   during childbirth, 183, 238–39
   cost of, 132
   how it works, 131, 183
   insurance for, 132
   during labor, 183
   prenatal, 131–32, 238–39
   research on, 131
   to speed up labor onset, 239
afterbirth. *See* placenta
age, maternal, 22–23, 41
airplane travel, 74–75
alcohol use
   aversion to alcohol during
      pregnancy, 97–98
   and BBT charting, 25
   and birth defects, 97
   and breastfeeding, 312–13
   and conception, 5–7, 11

debates about, 97–99
fetal alcohol syndrome, 63, 97
and miscarriage, 34, 64
and teratogens, 96–97
Allergan, 103
aluminum chloride hexahydrate, 108t
American Academy of Pediatrics
   (AAP), 327–28
American College of Obstetricians
   and Gynecologists, 180
AMH (anti-Mullerian hormone), 22
amniocentesis, 70, 136–37, 139–42
amniotic fluid, function of, 141
amniotomy, 241–42
amygdala, 338
ancestry testing, 46
anemia, hemolytic, 142
anemia, postpartum, 292–93, 313
aneuploidy, 35
anti-Mullerian hormone (AMH), 22
Apgar, Virginia, 251–52
Apgar scores, 88, 181, 251–52
aromatherapy, 182–84
ARRIVE study, 241
ART (Assisted Reproductive
   Technology) report, 45

aspirin, 270
autism, 12, 97

baby blues, 267, 270, 291. *See also*
    postpartum depression
baby budget, 15–19
Baby Killer report, 320
baby registry, 18, 157–61
bacterial vaginosis, 24
basal body temperature (BBT), 25
bathing during pregnancy, 64–65
Baumrind, Diane, 334
BBT (basal body temperature), 25
beta-hCG tests, 32
birth. *See* childbirth
birth centers, 78, 80, 86, 214
birth certificate, 223
birth class, 214–15
birth control
    breastfeeding as, 293–94
    IUD, 9, 294
    postpartum, 268, 282, 293–94
    quitting, 3, 5, 9–10
birth defects
    causes, 34–35, 73, 96–97, 99, 106,
        111
    of the heart, 12
    and maternal age, 22
    preventing, 12*t*
    screening, 6, 138–39, 141
birth spacing, 345–46
Bishop score, 241
bleeding
    from a fallopian-tube rupture, 40
    of gums, 151, 154
    implantation, 30, 35
    during IVF, 44
    postpartum, 267–68, 272–73
    spotting during labor, 240, 244
    spotting during ovulation, 11

blood pressure, 151, 211, 232–33,
    264*t*, 278
blood volume, 120
BMI (body mass index), 112
body dysmorphia, 283
Botox, 96, 102–3, 102*t*
Braxton Hicks contractions, 206,
    242, 245
breastfeeding
    as birth control, 293–94
    and bottle feeding, 317–20, 342
    breast maintenance, 307–8
    and breast size, 300
    complications, 297–98
    after C-sections, 254, 299, 305,
        310–11
    diet and vitamins, 292–93
    difficulty with, troubleshooting,
        309–10
    and doulas, 300
    duration, 297–98
    vs. formula feeding, xxi, 160, 298,
        301, 308, 320
    freezing milk, 315–16
    frequency, 297, 302–3
    gear for, 160
    and getting your old body back,
        282–83
    how it works, 302–5, *303–4*
    how-to, 307
    immunity benefits, 301
    and IQ, 301
    lactation consultants (LCs),
        299–300
    lactation support, xx
    low milk production, 309, 312–13
    mastitis, 276, 278, 309, 316
    and milk banks, 322–23
    milk supply, 301, 308–9, 312–14,
        344

myths about, 299–302
night feedings, 279
nipple pain, 275–76
nutritional and caloric
    requirements, 312
painful, 304–5
partner's role, 305, 317, 342
positions, 305, 306
and postpartum depression, 298
pros and cons, 299
pumping at work, xx, 221, 344
pumps and pumping, 160,
    220–22, 269, 314–16
resources at work, xx
and rooming-in, 194
schedule for, 302
tongue-tie, 298, 309–10
torticollis, 310
weaning, 316–17
and weight loss, 300–301
wet nurses, 309
breast tenderness/swelling, 52, 60
breech birth, 237–39, 242, 249
Brown, Louise, 44
budgeting, 15–16

caffeine, 11, 116–17
calorie intake, 292
cannabidiol (CBD), 100–101
cannabis, 100–102, 178
carbon monoxide, 96
carpal tunnel syndrome, 207
cat litter box, 71–72
CBD (cannabidiol), 100–101
CCHD (congenital heart defect)
    test, 253–54
CDC (Centers for Disease Control
    and Prevention), 45, 118
cell-free DNA (cfDNA) screening,
    136

cell phone use, 72
Centers for Disease Control and
    Prevention (CDC), 45, 118
certified midwives (CMs), 86
certified nurse-midwives (CNMs),
    86
certified professional midwives
    (CPMs), 86
cervical mucus, 24–28, 43, 244
cervical sweep, 240
cesarean section. See C-sections
Chicago Lying-In Hospital, 77
childbirth. See also C-sections;
    labor; newborn care; prenatal
    care; recovery after childbirth
    acupuncture during, 183, 238–39
    aromatherapy, 182–84
    breech birth, 237–39, 242, 249
    epidural, 177–82, 238, 250–51
    episiotomy, 78
    fathers in the delivery room, 77
    fear of, 235–36
    forceps use, 78, 180
    "golden hour" after, 251–54
    history of, xix
    in hospitals vs. at home, 78–80
    hypnobirthing, 184
    Lamaze, 184–85
    massage, 185
    maternal mortality rates, xix,
        77–78
    medications for, 176, 178–79,
        186
    modesty during, 255–56
    narcotics (opioids), 182
    nitrous oxide, 179, 181–82
    overview, 235–36
    perineal tearing, 177
    physiological limits of, xiv
    postpartum stay after, 254–58

childbirth (*cont.*)
  preferences (*see* childbirth
    preferences)
  speeding up labor onset, 239–40
  TENS (transcutaneous electrical
    nerve stimulation), 187
  vaginal, and due date, 236–37
    (*see also* due date)
  vaginal, postpartum prep kit for,
    233
  water immersion, 186–87
  when it doesn't go as planned,
    254–58
childbirth preferences
  checklist/outline, 194–98
  "natural," xix, 176
  pain management, medical,
    178–82
  pain management, nonmedical,
    176–78, 182–87
  vs. plans, 175–76
Childbirth Without Fear
  (Dick-Read), 176
childcare
  au pair, 230–31
  costs, 15–16
  day care, 17, 226–27, 344
  family childcare centers, 227–28
  by family members, 17
  gender inequality of, 280
  jealousy of caregivers, 343
  nanny, 17, 228–30
  planning, 225–26
  staying at home, 231–32
  transitioning to, 341, 344
children, cost of raising, 15–18
chimerism, 345
China, 281
Chinese birth table, 69
Chinese medicine. *See* acupuncture

chlamydia, 191
chloroform, 178
choline, 13*t*
chorionic villus sampling (CVS), 70,
  136–42, 144–45
cigarettes. *See* smoking
circumcision, 192–93, 253
Clomid, 42
CMV (cytomegalovirus), 73
coffee, 116–17
college fund for newborn, 19
compound interest, 19
computer use, 72, 129
conception. *See also* fertility;
    infertility; ovulation;
    pregnancy; prenatal care; sex;
    sperm health/quality
  and age, 22
  and alcohol use, 5–7
  anxiety and stress about, 5, 29
  baby budget, creating, 15–19
  birth control, stopping, 9–10
  and birth defects, 6, 12, 34–35
  caffeine consumption, 6, 11
  checklist, 48
  drug use, 5–6
  due date calculation, 65
    (*see also* due date)
  eggs, quantity vs. quality, 22
  fertile window for, 10, 23–25, 27,
    42–43
  fertility testing, 7–8
  finances, 15–19
  genetic carrier screenings, 8–9
  via IVF, 9, 32, 44–45, 47
  lifestyle and health, 3, 4–5, 11
  medical checkup before, 5–7
  meiosis, 34–35
  menstrual cycles, 10–11, 23–24,
    237 (*see also* LMP)

overview, 2
parenting and life expectations,
    3–5
and parenting goals/philosophy,
    19–20
partner's role, 4–5
patience, 5
prenatal vitamins, 12–14
problems conceiving
    (*see* infertility)
and resentment, 3–4
smoking, 5
congenital heart defect (CCHD)
    test, 253–54
constipation
    of baby, 321, 332
    of mother, 13, 61–62, 205, 240,
        274–75, 288, 290, 293
CoQ10, 13
cord prolapse, 239, 242
cortisol, 7–8, 128
cravings, 59, 111, 157
crib standards, 328
Cruise, Tom, 112
C-sections
    belly binding and wrapping after,
        288
    and birth spacing, 345–46
    breastfeeding after, 254, 299, 305,
        310–11
    for breech babies, 238–39
    doulas and incidence of, 88
    for emergency deliveries, 79
    for failure to progress, 249
    fear of, 235
    frequency, 80, 249
    and home births, 79
    incisions/scars from, 250–51
    medical preferences for, 188,
        210–11

for placenta previa, 238
postpartum prep kit for, 233
postpartum stay after, 254
preferences for, 196–97
pre-scheduled, 235, 249–50
pros and cons, 249–50
recovery, 265–66
for sexual assault/abuse sufferers,
    249
vaginal birth after, 250
what to expect, 250–51, 257–58
CVS (chorionic villus sampling), 70,
    136–42, 144–45
cycling, 5, 40
cystic fibrosis, 8
cytomegalovirus (CMV), 73

dairy foods, 116
data tracking
    anxiety due to, 308–9
    fertility, 26–27
    menstrual cycle, 10–11, 52
dates (fruit, not social life), 240
D&C (dilation and curettage),
    37–38
DEA (Drug Enforcement Agency),
    100
deep vein thrombosis (DVT), 74–75
dehydroepiandrosterone (DHEA),
    7–8
DeLee, Joseph, 77–78
deli meats, 117–18
delivery. *See* childbirth
depression, 54, 91–92, 128, 207.
    See also postpartum depression
DHEA (dehydroepiandrosterone),
    7–8
diabetes, 34, 78–79, 111, 143–44.
    See also gestational diabetes
diaper rash, 332

diapers
    cost, 15–17, 18*t*
    number needed, 159
    and poop, 331–32
    tracking, 301, 308
diarrhea during labor, 243
diastasis recti, 169, 172–74, 286–88
Dick-Read, Grantly, 177
    Childbirth Without Fear, 176
diet and nutrition
    for breastfeeding, 292–93
    before conception, 5
    cooking, help with, 116
    dairy products, 116
    eating for two, 112
    first trimester, 111–12, 114–19
    foods to avoid, 117–19
    fruits, 115
    grains, 116
    and menstrual cycles, 11
    during postpartum recovery,
        292–93
    proteins, 115
    vegetables, 115
    vitamins and supplements, 5,
        12–14, 292–93
dilation and curettage (D&C),
    37–38
dizziness, 40, 66, 154
Donald, Ian, 134
Dona.org, 89
doulas
    benefits of, 88, 90–91
    birth philosophy of, 88
    credentials for, 89
    fees for, 90
    find/choosing, 89–90
    function/definition of, xiv,
        87–88
    growing use of, 88

postpartum home visits, 89,
    281–82
Down syndrome, 22, 136–38
drinking. *See* alcohol use
Drug Enforcement Agency (DEA),
    100
drugs
    narcotics (opioids), 182
    for pain management during
        labor, 178–82
    recreational, 5–7, 34, 41, 96,
        100–102, 178 (*see also specific
        drugs*)
due date, 52, 65, 135, 236–37, 254
DVT (deep vein thrombosis),
    74–75

e-cigarettes, 99
E. coli, 118, 191
ectopic pregnancy, 39–40, 44
ECV (external cephalic version),
    238
EDD (estimated due date), 52, 65,
    237
edema, 207–9
Edwards syndrome (trisomy 18),
    144–45
electromagnetic waves, 72
embryologists, 44–45
endocrine-disrupting chemicals, 40
endometriosis, 8, 40
Environmental Working Group, 97
Epidiolex, 101
epidural, 238, 250–51
epidural (anesthetic), 177–82
episiotomy, 78
essential oils, 109*t*, 183–84
estimated due date (EDD), 52, 65,
    237
estradiol, 7–8, 41

estrogen, 23–24, 62, 68, 190, 291, 294, 303
exercise
  for abs, 287–88
  and DR (diastasis recti), 173, 286–88
  first trimester, 120–28, *123–27*
  foam rolling, 129–30
  high-impact activities to avoid, 120
  Kegels, 167, 286
  and menstrual cycles, 11
  pelvic floor, 169–71, 284
  Pilates, 128, 169, 287
  postpartum, 283–86
  strength training, 122–28, *123–27*
  walking, to speed up labor onset, 239
  yoga, 64, 122, 169
external cephalic version (ECV), 238
eye drops for newborns, 191–92, 253

facials, 102*t*, 104
fainting, 40, 66, 151, 154
fallopian tube, rupture of, 39–40
family practice physicians, 87
fatigue, 57–58, 272
FDA (Food and Drug Administration), xxi, 43, 101, 103, 137, 321
female pelvic medicine and reconstructive surgery (FPMRS), 290
feminine hygiene products, 24–25
fentanyl, 100, 182
fertility. *See also* infertility
  and age, 22–23
  number and quality of eggs, 22
  sensors for, 26–27

testing for, 7–8
tracking of (*see* ovulation)
window of, 10, 23–25, 27, 42–43
Fertility Rules (Schrock), xviii, xxi
fetal alcohol syndrome, 63, 97
fetal microchimerism, 345
50/30/20 budgeting rule, 15–16
finances, 15–19
Finland, 158
first-time mothers
  age, 22
  due date, 237
  home vs. hospital births, 78
  induced labor for, 241
  lightening, 243
  perineal pain/tearing, 288–89
  quickening (feeling first fetal movement), 67
first trimester. *See also* prenatal care
  acupuncture, 131–32
  alcohol, 63–64, 97–99
  bathing, 64–65
  brain changes, 68–69
  caffeine, 116–17
  cannabis, 100–102
  care team, history of, 77–79
  care team, processing data from, 92–93
  checklist, 146
  and CMV, 73
  cosmetic procedures, 102–6, 102*t*, 106–9*t*
  diet, 111–12, 114–19 (*see also* diet and nutrition)
  differences between pregnancies, 50–51
  exercise, 64, 120–28, *123–27*
  FAQs, 63–75
  fetal growth, by month, 52–53
  first prenatal appointment, 53, 64

first trimester (*cont.*)
  foods to avoid, 117–19
  gender prediction, 68–69, 136
  genetic testing, 138–42
  illness and medications during,
    72–73
  and infertility anxiety, 73–74
  ingredients to avoid, 106–9t
  massage, 128–29
  maternal experience, by month,
    52–54
  micromanaging, 50–51
  overheating, 64–65, 121
  overview, 50–51
  pain management, 128–32
  partner's role, 55–56
  placenta, functions of, 95–96
  quickening (first fetal movement
    felt), 67–68
  saunas, 64–65
  screening/testing (*see* prenatal
    screening/testing)
  sex, 65–66
  skin-color changes, 68
  smoking/vaping, 99
  symptoms, lack of, 53, 66
  symptoms and solutions, 54–55,
    57–62
  teratogens, avoiding, 96–97
  travel, 74–75
  uterus, function of, 95
  weight gain, recommended,
    112–13, 112t
  weight loss, 66
  when to share news, 66–67
  and the work environment, 67
flexible spending account (FSA),
  16–17
foam rolling, 128–32
folate, 12t, 13

Foley catheter, 241
folic acid/B9/folate, 12t
follicle-stimulating hormone (FSH),
  131
Food and Drug Administration.
  See FDA
food aversions and cravings, 59, 111,
  157
food-poisoning culprits, 117–18
foot growth, 71
forceps delivery, 78, 180
formaldehyde, 107t
formula
  bottles for, 160, 317, 319–20
  vs. breastfeeding, xxi, 160, 298,
    301, 308, 320
  vs. breast milk, quality of,
    320–21
  cost, 15, 17, 18t
  history and popularity of, 320
  types, 321
fourth trimester. *See* postpartum
  period
FPMRS (female pelvic medicine
  and reconstructive surgery),
  290
fragile X syndrome, 8
French parenting, 334–35
fruits, 115
FSA (flexible spending account),
  16–17
FSH (follicle-stimulating hormone),
  131
fundal height, 83, 204

galactagogues, 312
gamete donation, 45–46
gardening, 71–72
gas and bloating, 58
Gaskin, Ina May, 176–77

GBS (group B strep) test, 133, 144–45
GDF15 (hormone), 66
GDM. *See* gestational diabetes
gender prediction, 69–70, 136
genetic inheritance, 8
genetic testing, 8–9, 46, 140–42, 252–53. *See also* amniocentesis
gestational carrier/surrogate, 44, 46–47
gestational diabetes, 82*t*, 133, 143–44, 241
gingivitis, pregnancy, 151, 154
GLP-agonists, 111
glucose screening, 82*t*, 143–44
glycolic acid, 104
gonorrhea, 191
grains, whole, 116
group B strep (GBS) test, 133, 144–45
gummy vitamins and supplements, 14
gynecology, 80–81

hair loss, 269, 271
hair treatments, 102*t*, 104–5
hCG (human chorionic gonadotropin), 31–32, 39, 69
health insurance, 16
health savings account (HSA), 16–17
heartbeat, fetal, 36, 53, 56, 83, 135
heartburn and reflux, 58–59, 111
hemolytic anemia, 142
hemorrhoids, 205, 275
hepatitis, 104, 322
hepatitis B vaccine for newborns, 191, 253
herpes, 193, 242
HIV, 104, 193, 322
home births, 78–80

HoP (Holder pasteurization), 322
hormones. *See also* estrogen; progesterone
at-home tests, 7
cortisol, 7–8, 128
DHEA, 7–8
estradiol, 7–8, 41
FSH, 131
GDF15, 66
hCG, 31–32, 39, 69
LH, 25–26, 131
testosterone, 7–8, 42
hot tubs during pregnancy, 64–65
HPO (hypothalamus-pituitary-ovarian) axis, 131
HPV, 193
HSA (health savings account), 16–17
human chorionic gonadotropin (hCG), 31–32, 69
hydroquinone, 106*t*
hyperemesis gravidarum, 66
hypertension, 78–79, 151. *See also* blood pressure
hyperthermia, 64
hypothalamus-pituitary-ovarian (HPO) axis, 131

ibuprofen, 72, 116–17, 269–70
ICI (intracervical insemination), 29, 43
incontinence
postpartum, 169, 267, 274, 287, 289–91
urinary, 247, 249–50, 274
infant mortality, 158, 238
infertility
and age, 41
anxiety about, 73–74
causes of, 40

infertility (*cont.*)
  clinics for, finding, 45
  gamete donation, 45–46
  gestational carrier/surrogate, 44,
    46–47
  IUI (intrauterine insemination),
    29, 43–44, 47
  IVF (in vitro fertilization), 9, 32,
    44–45, 47
  of men, xxi, 4–5, 23, 34, 40
  overview, 40–42
  rates of, xxi, 40, 42
  secondary, xxi, 33
  testing, 41–42
  treatments, 42–47
  when to seek help, 40–41
  of women, 5, 40–41
injectable cosmetic procedures,
    102t, 103
insomnia, 152
insurance
  for acupuncture, 132
  adding baby to your policy, 224
  categories of items covered, 18t
  changing coverage outside
    open enrollment, 16
  for doulas, 90
  for home births and birth centers,
    80
  for midwife services, 80, 86
  for pelvic floor therapy, 169, 286
  for a postnatal nurse, 281
  for prenatal testing, 134
  what's covered by a standard
    health plan, 16
intracervical insemination (ICI),
    29, 43
intravaginal insemination (IVI), 29, 43
in vitro fertilization. *See* IVF
iodine, 13t

iron, 12t, 13, 292–93, 322
IUDs, 9, 294
IUI (intrauterine insemination), 29,
    43–44, 47
IVF (in vitro fertilization), 9, 32,
    44–45, 47
IVI (intravaginal insemination), 29,
    43

Jessner solution, 104

Kegels, 167, 286
kitty litter, 71–72

labor. *See also* childbirth
  acupuncture during, 183
  the baby drops (lightening), 243
  back labor, 256
  bloody show/spotting, 244
  Braxton Hicks contractions
    (false labor), 206, 242, 245
  cervical changes, 243
  diarrhea, 243
  dilation, 243
  early signs, 242–45
  induction, 241–42
  memory of pain during, 178,
    235–36
  modesty during, 255–56
  mucus plug, 244
  pain management, medical,
    178–82
  pain management, nonmedical,
    176–78, 182–87
  somatic pain, 246
  speeding up onset, 239–40
  stage 1 (early/active/transitional),
    245–47
  stage 2 (pushing/crowning),
    247–48

stage 3 (placenta delivery), 188, 248–49, 251
visceral pain, 246
water breaks, 244–45
weight loss/stabilization during, 244
when to go to hospital/birthing center, 246
labor nurses, xiv
lactational amenorrhea, 293
lactic acid, 104
Lamaze, 184–85
Lamaze, Fernand, 184
laptop use, 72, 129
laser hair removal, 102t, 103
leg cramps, 151–53
LGBTQ couples, gestational carrier/ surrogacy for, 46–47
LH (luteinizing hormone), 25–26, 131
Liebig, Justus von, 320
linea nigra, 68, 70, 151–52
listeria, 118
LMP (last menstrual period), 10, 52, 65, 96, 237
lochia, 267–68, 294
luteinizing hormone (LH), 25–26, 131
lycopene, 13
lying on your back during pregnancy, 71

makeup, 105–9
manicures/pedicures, 102t, 105
marijuana/cannabis, 100–102, 178
massage
during first trimester, 128–29
during labor, 185
perineal, 171–72
mastitis, 276, 278, 309, 316

maternal-fetal medicine, xiv
maternal-fetal medicine specialists (MFMs), 80, 84–85
maternity clothes, 17, 157, 162–66
matrescence, 338
Mayan birth table, 70
meconium, 245, 308, 331–32
Medela, 220
Medicaid, 90
medical checkups
before conception, 5–7
postpartum, 169, 282, 287
prenatal, 53, 64, 82–83t
medications
for childbirth, 176, 178–79, 186
for illnesses in first trimester, 72–73
meiotic errors, 34–35
melanocytes, 68
melasma, 68
melatonin, 330
membrane sweep, 240
Mendel, Gregor, 8
menopause, 291
menstrual cycles, 10–11, 23–24, 26, 237. See also LMP
methotrexate, 40
MFMs (maternal-fetal medicine specialists), 80, 84–85
microcephaly, 73
midwives, xiv
acupuncture training, 183
certified, 86
female vs. male, 77
history of midwifery, 77
hospital-based, 86
insurance coverage for, 80, 86
limits of practice, 86
medical training/certification levels of, 85–86
vs. ob-gyns, 79–80, 85–86

midwives (*cont.*)
  reputation of, 78
  resurgence of, 85
mifepristone, 36–37
milk banks, 322
minimum viable registry, 158
miscarriages
  and alcohol use, 34
  causes of, 31, 34
  chemical pregnancies, 31
  chromosomal abnormality as a
    cause of, 22, 31, 34–35
  dilation and curettage (D&C)
    after the ninth week, 37
  expectant management of, 36
  feeling like a failure, 34
  fertility after, 38
  first-trimester, 31, 36
  frequency of, 31, 34
  grief/healing after, 37–39
  with IVF, 44
  legislation affecting medical care
    for, 36
  and lifestyle, 34
  missed/silent, 36
  myths about, 34–38
  overview, 33–34
  recurrent, 35
  resolution of, 36–37
  sex after, 37
  signs of, 35–36
  stillbirth, 33, 241
  terms for, 33
  therapy after, 38
  what to do during, 36
misoprostol, 36–37
morning sickness, 12, 31, 52–55, 57,
    66, 111, 149
morphine, 178, 182
multiple births, 44–45, 112, 238, 249

naming the baby, 222–24
naproxen, 269–70
narcotics (opioids), 182
National Institutes of Health (NIH),
    xxi
"natural" pregnancy and childbirth,
    xix, 176
Needham, Orwell H., 220
Netherlands, 281
newborn care
  Apgar test, 88, 181, 251–52
  bathing, 251, 253
  circumcision, 192–93, 253
  congenital heart defect (CCHD)
    test, 253–54
  cord blood banking, 189–90
  cord clamping, 188, 252
  eye drops, 191–92, 253
  genetic testing, 252–53
  hearing test, 253
  heel-stick test, 252–53
  hepatitis B vaccine, 191
  preferences for, 197
  rooming-in vs. nursery, 194
  vitamin K shot, 192, 253
newborns
  behavior of, understanding,
    325–26
  bonding, 262, 278–79, 304
  bottle feeding, 317–20, 342
  clothing and gear for,
    157–61
  colic, 331
  co-sleeping, 328
  crying, 330–31
  cuteness of, 325
  developmental percentiles/
    milestones, 333
  donor milk, 322–23
  epidural's effects on, 181

feeding time, overview of, 297–98
  (*see also* breastfeeding)
formula feeding (*see* formula)
growth, by month, 267–68
hearing, 326
keeping warm, 326
Moro (startle) reflex, 328
online identity of, 296
overstimulation, 330
pacifiers, 331
poop and diapers, 331–32
premature, 99, 103, 322
sleeping, 327–28
socializing by, 343–44
swaddling, 328–30, 329
taste, sense of, 326
umbilical cord stump, 326
vision, 326
visitors' handling of, 295
weight fluctuations, 308–9, 311
nicotine. *See* smoking
night sweats, 270–71
NIH (National Institutes of Health),
  xxi
911 service, 264*t*
nipple pain, 275–76
nipple stimulation, 239
nitrous oxide, 179, 181–82
nose, growth of, 71
nose, stuffy, 153
nutrition. *See* diet and nutrition
nutritionists, 119, 143

obesity, 40, 111–12, 299
ob-gyns, 79–85, 82–83*t*
obstetrics
  definition of, 80
  evolution and overview of, xiv,
    77–78, 178
  traditional, 177

omega-3 fatty acids, 13*t*
ovarian failure, premature, 22
overheating, 64–65, 121, 151
ovulation
  basal body temperature (BBT), 25
  cervical mucus, 24–28
  fertility sensors, 26–27
  how it works, 23–27
  ovulation predictor kits (OPKs),
    25–26
  postpartum, 268, 293–94
  spotting during, 11
  stopped via birth control, 9
  and timing of sex, 23–24
  waiting for signs of pregnancy,
    29–30
oxytocin, 184, 239, 241–42, 249,
  299–300, 303–4

padsicle recipe, 289–90
pain management
  first trimester, 128–32
  medical, 178–82
  nonmedical, 176–78, 182–87
Papyrus Ebers, 309
parabens, 109*t*
parental leave, 17, 224–25, 237
parenting
  advice/criticism about, 95, 263,
    295
  cost of raising children, 15
  division of labor, 4
  goals/philosophy/styles, 19–20,
    333–36
  as transformative, 3–4
partner's role
  breastfeeding, 305
  conception, 4–5
  first trimester, 55–56
  postpartum period, 263, 277–80

partner's role (*cont.*)
    prenatal vitamins, 13
    third trimester, 210–11, 214
paternity testing, 141
PCOS (polycystic ovary syndrome),
    8, 24, 26, 43
pediatricians, 219–20, 282,
    333
peeing, frequent, 61, 69
pelvic floor, 167–71, *168*, 283–84,
    286, 290
perinatologists, 80
perineal and vaginal tearing, 177,
    286, 288–90
perineal discomfort, 273
perineal massage, 171–72
personal care products, 105–9
phthalates, 107*t*
piercings, 102*t*, 104
pills, birth control.
    See birth control
Pitocin, 239, 241–42, 255–57
placenta
    as a barrier, 96, 103, 182
    consumption of (placentophagy),
        190–91
    delivery of, 248–49, 251
    diagnostic testing via, 139
    functions of, 95–96, 190
    and the umbilical cord, 188
placenta previa, 78–79, 238, 242
PMS symptoms, 10
polycystic ovary syndrome (PCOS),
    8, 24, 26, 43
POP (pelvic organ prolapse), 169,
    286, 290–91
postpartum depression (PPD)
    maternal, 191, 282, 291–92,
        298
    paternal, 277–78

postpartum period, xviii, xx. *See also*
    recovery after childbirth
    advice/criticism during, 263,
        295
    baby blues, 267, 270
    baby's growth, by month,
        267–68
    birth control, 268, 282, 293–94
    bleeding, 267–68, 272–73
    bonding, 262, 278–79, 304
    constipation, 274–75
    diastasis recti, 286–88
    division of labor during, 3–4
    fatigue, 272
    hair loss, 269, 271
    hemorrhoids, 205, 275
    incontinence, 169, 267, 274, 287,
        289–91
    mastitis, 276, 278, 309, 316
    maternal changes, by month,
        267–69
    mom guilt, 279, 338–39, 342–44
    mommy shaming, xx
    mothering behaviors, 338
    night sweats, 270–71
    nipple pain, 275–76
    overview, 262–63
    ovulation, 268, 293–94
    partner's role, 263, 277–80
    pelvic floor, 283–84, 286, 290
    perineal discomfort, 273
    postpartum prep kit, 232–33
    sex, 268, 280, 290, 293
    six-week checkup, 169, 282, 287
    sleep deprivation, 269, 278
    symptoms and solutions,
        269–76
    transitions, overview, 337–39
    uterine contractions, 269–70,
        283

visitors, 294–96
weight fluctuations, 266
work, return to, 339–42
preeclampsia, 257, 278
pregnancy
average length, xxii
chemical, 31
complications, xiv–xv (*see also* breech birth)
early signs, 30 (*see also* morning sickness)
ectopic, 39–40, 44
FAQs, 63–75
illness during, 72–73
low- vs. high-risk, 78–79
lying on your back during, 71
mood changes during, 91–92
"natural," xix, 176
parenting advice during, 95
seat belt use, 74
sex during, 65–66, 239
stages (*see* first trimester; second trimester; third trimester)
stomach sleeping during, 70
stress of, 55, 151
termination of, 37–38, 145
tests to detect, 30–32
as transformative for women, 4
waiting for signs, 29
when to share news, 66–67
pregnancy brain, 68–69, 150
pregnancy gingivitis, 151, 154
pregorexia, 283
prenatal care. *See also* doulas; midwives
acupuncture, 131–32
appointment/testing schedule, 82–83*t*
family practice physicians, 87
group care, 87

midwives, 79–80
ob-gyns, 79–85, 82–83*t*
pelvic exam, 83
pelvic floor therapy, 169, 286, 290
telemedicine, 79
therapists, 91–92
prenatal screening/testing
amniocentesis, 70, 136–37, 139–42
benefits and risks of, 133–34
cfDNA (cell-free DNA), 136–38
CVS (chorionic villus sampling), 70, 136–42, 144–45
GBS (group B strep) test, 133, 144–45
glucose, 82*t*, 143–44
NIPS (noninvasive), 70, 136–38
nuchal translucency screening, 135–36
quadruple, 138–39
rhesus (Rh) factor blood test, 142–43
stress of, 134
ultrasounds, 65, 70, 134–36
prenatal vitamins, 12–14
progesterone, 23–24, 26, 58–61, 68, 128, 190, 303
prolactin, 293, 303–4, 312
PROM (premature rupture of the membranes), 244
prostaglandins, 239–43
proteins, 115

quadruple screening (quad screen), 138–39
Quetelet, Adolphe, 112
quickening (first fetal movement felt), 67–68, 149

radiation, 135
Ramzi method, 68–69
recovery after childbirth. *See also*
    postpartum depression
baby blues, 267, 270, 291
belly binding and wrapping,
    288
complications, 286–91
diastasis recti, 169, 172–74,
    286–88
diet, 292–93
doula's home visit, 281–82
exercise, 283–86
getting your old body back,
    282–83
mental health, 291–92
overview, 281–82
pelvic organ prolapse (POP), 169,
    286, 290–91
perineal and vaginal tearing, 177,
    286, 288–90
postpartum checkup, 282
support system, 281–82
warning signs, 264–66, 264*t*
reflux and heartburn, 58–59,
    111
relaxin, 71, 121–22
reproductive endocrinologist, 41
research limitations, xxi–xxii
restless legs, 152–53, 208
retinoids, 106
Rh-negative blood type, 37,
    142–43
rib-cage expansion, 71, 121–22
round ligament pain, 155
Royal Oldham Hospital
    (United Kingdom), 44

salicylic acid, 104, 106, 108*t*
salmonella, 118

SART (Society for Assisted
    Reproductive Technology),
    45
saunas, 5, 29, 64–65
Schmorl, Georg, 345
Schrock, Leslie
    Fertility Rules, xviii, xxi
Schwarzenegger, Arnold, 112
sciatica, 128, 209
sclerotherapy, 102*t*, 103
secondhand smoke, 99
second trimester. *See also*
    prenatal care
baby gear/registry, 157–62
checklist, 199
diastasis recti, 169, 172–74
exercise in (*see* exercise)
fetal growth, by month, *149*,
    149–51
maternal experience, by month,
    149–51
maternity clothes, 157,
    162–66
overview, 148
pelvic floor, 167–71, *168*
perineal massage, 171–72
planning for childbirth
    (*see* childbirth preferences)
quickening (first fetal movement
    felt), 149
shopping/registry list, 157–61
symptoms and solutions,
    151–55
selenium, 13
sex
    after a D&C, 37–38
    douching and lubricants, 29
    frequency, 27–28
    lying on your back after,
        28–29

after a miscarriage, 37
positions, 28
postpartum, 268, 280, 290, 293
during pregnancy, 65–66, 239
to speed up labor onset, 239
timed, 29, 42–43
sexual-abuse survivors, 83, 249
sexually transmitted diseases (STDs), 24, 46, 191, 193. *See also* *specific diseases*
shopping/registry list, 18, 157–61
sickle cell disease, 8
SIDS (sudden infant death syndrome), 99, 328–29
Simpson, James, 178
single parents, gestational carrier/surrogacy for, 45–47
skin changes, 68, 151–52
sleep
    co-sleeping with newborns, 328
    and menstrual cycles, 11
    of newborns, 327–28
    postpartum deprivation of, 269, 278
    stomach sleeping during pregnancy, 70
    twilight, 178–79
smell, heightened sense of, 62
smoking, 5, 25, 34, 40–41, 99, 301
Snow, John, 178
Society for Assisted Reproductive Technology (SART), 45
South Korea, 281
sperm health/quality, 4–5, 7–8, 13, 23, 27–28, 34, 40, 43
spina bifida, 138
spotting. *See* bleeding

STDs (sexually transmitted diseases), 24, 46, 191, 193. *See also* *specific diseases*
stem cells, 189
steroids, 5
stillbirth, 33, 241. *See also* miscarriages
stomach sleeping during pregnancy, 70
strep, group B, 133, 144
Streptococcus agalactiae, 190–91
stress, emotional
    aromatherapy for, 183
    and conception, 5, 29
    and constipation, 62
    menstrual cycle affected by, 11
    and miscarriage, 34
    of pregnancy, 55, 151
    of prenatal testing, 134
    recreational drugs for, 100
    of returning to work, 341–42
    sensors for tracking, 26–27
    and sperm count, 40
stretch marks, 69
stuffy nose, 153
sudden infant death syndrome (SIDS), 99, 328–29
sunscreens, chemical, 108*t*
syphilis, 193

tattoos, 101*t*, 104
Tay-Sachs disease, 8, 141
TCA (trichloroacetic acid), 104
tea, 116–17
telemedicine, 79
TENS (transcutaneous electrical nerve stimulation), 187

teratogens, 96–97. *See also* alcohol use; drugs; smoking
testosterone, 7–8, 42
thalidomide, xxi
THC (tetrahydrocannabinol), 100–101
therapy
  aromatherapy, 182–84
  emotional/psychological, 91–92
  after miscarriage, 38
  pelvic floor, 169, 286, 290
  sclerotherapy, 102*t*, 103
third trimester. *See also* childbirth; prenatal care
  acupuncture during, 238–39
  birth class, 214–15
  breast pump, registering for, 220–22
  checklist, 259
  childcare planning (*see* childcare)
  fetal growth, by month, *204*, 204–6
  hospital/birthing center tour and preregistering, 215–16
  kick counts, 202
  maternal experience, by month, 204–6
  naming the baby, 222–24
  overview, 202–3, 213
  packing your bag, 216–19
  parental-leave arrangements, 224–25
  partner's role, 210–11, 214
  pediatrician, choosing, 219–20
  postpartum prep kit, 232–33
  strangers touching your belly, 203
  symptoms and solutions, 206–9

thyroid, 283
toxoplasmosis, 71–72, 118
transcutaneous electrical nerve stimulation (TENS), 187
transverse abdominis (TVA), 287
travel, 74–75
trichloroacetic acid (TCA), 104
trimester zero. *See* conception
trisomy 18 (Edwards syndrome), 144–45
TVA (transverse abdominis), 287
twilight sleep, 178–79

ultrasounds, 65, 70, 134–36
umbilical cord, 188–90, 239, 242, 251–52, 326
uterus
  contractions of, 269–70, 283
  function of, 23, 95
  size of, 95
UTIs (urinary tract infections), 69, 193

vaccines for newborns, 191, 253
vaping, 99
varicocele, 40
varicose veins, 103
vegetables, 115
vernix caseosa, 150, 205–6
Victoria, Queen, 178
vitamin K shot for newborns, 192, 253
vitamins and supplements, 5, 12–14, 292–93

walking, to speed up labor onset, 239

water-immersion childbirth, 186–87
water/liquid consumption, 11, 26, 61, 69, 74, 116–17, 121, 245
weight gain, 112t, 113, 206, 244, 283
work
first trimester, and the work environment, 67

pumping breast milk at, xx, 221, 344
resources at, xx
returning to, xx, 221, 339–42, 344

yeast infections, 24
yoga during pregnancy, 64

zinc, 13

ABOUT THE AUTHOR

LESLIE SCHROCK is an author, entrepreneur, and investor working at the convergence of health and technology. She is the author of *Bumpin'* and *Fertility Rules*. Leslie was named one of *Fast Company*'s Most Creative People in Business, and her writing and other work has been featured in *The Economist, Time, GQ, Fortune, Entrepreneur, Wired,* and the *New York Times,* and on CNBC and NPR. She lives in Brooklyn with her husband and two sons. Connect with Leslie at LeslieSchrock.com.